We Learn As We Grow

Books gives Healing Hands; Life makes Caring Hearts.

Dr Yogesh A Gupta

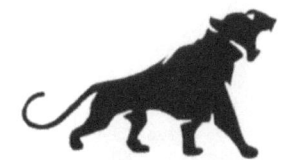

Ukiyoto Publishing

All global publishing rights are held by

Ukiyoto Publishing

Published in 2023

Content Copyright © Dr Yogesh A Gupta

ISBN 9789359207179

All rights reserved.
No part of this publication may be reproduced, transmitted, or stored in a retrieval system, in any form by any means, electronic, mechanical, photocopying, recording or otherwise, without the prior permission of the publisher.

The moral rights of the author have been asserted.

This book is sold subject to the condition that it shall not by way of trade or otherwise, be lent, resold, hired out or otherwise circulated, without the publisher's prior consent, in any form of binding or cover other than that in which it is published.

www.ukiyoto.com

Dedication

I dedicate this book to my professors, fellow colleagues and patients. I will like to specially thank my wife Dr. Geeta Gupta, daughters Manya and Arayna for the selfless support and love. I am deeply indebted to Dr. Rikin Shah, Dr. Urmit Shah, Dr Harsh Desai and Dr. Atul Patel sir for all the sanity that they have provided to me. This book is for all the medical students who entered with a dream and then are left high and dry with things that were never taught to them. I will like to pray for Indian Healthcare system.

Preface

A middle-class boy with good studies got good marks in the 12th standard. His dreams got wings, and he entered medical education. Billions like him were told that this was the best way to serve humanity.

So he enters MBBS with glowing eyes. There were 100 more such eyes on day 1. Then the psychological tutoring starts. First day in the dissection room. Bodies with a pungent smell of preservatives lying naked on benches. Some benches had only hands, some had only legs, some had part of the abdomen, and some had the upper torso. As we entered, it was nauseating; a few collapsed at the sight and smell. The majority could not eat a single meal for a few days due to the residual smell in our whole body. It was a nightmare. But then, by the end of the week, all were enjoying the lessons, dissection, and their meals as well.

Then there were bones everywhere the skull, the largest bone, the smallest one, holes/openings in the skull, eye sockets, and pelvic bones. Few enjoyed naming unknown openings in the skull, and few had stories of bones placed with candles at home like in Ramsay Brothers movies. But almost everyone had a bone set to study in lockers or homes.

Every lesson taught the minutest details of the human body. From skeleton to chemical, from physiology to biology, we learned all that was taught to us. But frankly, few learned with zeal; rest all only cramped. None had time to understand. Exams we're always on the corner.

The second year brought higher education. Pharmacology was there, and so was microbiology. Molecules after molecules, group, subgroup, effects, side effects, pharmacokinetics, and dynamics we were being taught the elixir of all suffering. Learning them, we were thinking about how each molecule can cure every disease in the world. Finally, I will be the master of relief for humankind. Lesser I knew...

Microbiology told me about the real enemy of mankind. Their structure, their defense, their attack, and their final outcome. Learning them, each medical student thought, come what may, I will destroy them and save my patient. Lesser do they know...

Then we entered the den of real suffering. Medicine, surgery, gynecology, and so on Disease after disease how they came, how they presented, how they were diagnosed and treated. And also how they can kill or make one suffer—prognosis. But still, the end was happy, as every chapter said this therapy or that procedure could finish this disease.

Phew 5 and a half years of MBBS, and my eyes, ears, and hands are trained to see, hear, and understand the human body, sufferings, the enemy, and management. I am ready to treat. My name is Dr. Xyzabc.

To learn more, every student dreams of doing something after graduation, and so internal medicine was my calling. I entered the ward. All MBBS training appears blurry. It did help to survive the medical words, definitions, names of molecules, reports, and physiology, pathology, and microbiology. But that is it. Nothing of this mattered in final clinical practice. It was a new world that was not shown to us in MBBS. Terrified, we adjusted. With nowhere to go, we thrived. Stigmatized by being called a runaway, we survived.

The questions that came to mind were many.

Till date, I don't yet know when my education will come to an end. I am still confused about how important topics of medical practice were left out of the curriculum. I never understood why branded medicines are used in practice and not generic molecules, which we learned and practiced throughout medical education. If governments and policymakers knew we had to write brands only, why cheat us?

The topic of medical law and ethics was completely left out of the curriculum. How on earth is the subject that decides my way of practicing in real life not even touched upon? Why I was not taught what negligence is? I always thought chopping the wrong limb, leaving behind mops and instruments in the body, and giving treatment for typhoid despite having a malaria diagnosis were acts of negligence. I still don't understand how a possible failure in treatment, a possible death during treatment, a possible different differential diagnosis, or a possible common complication of a treatment can be caused by negligence. A health-illegal patient with the help of a lawyer can make any doctor's life full of court days and anxiety. Why was this not taught to me?

The predominant corporate hospitals are run by managers. Why did they not teach us that we would not be bosses in the hospital but slaves to these managers? They will decide what brands we use, which medicines we use in cases of government schemes, what investigations we order, whom to refer, and how we are to blame for bad food, high bills, and any ruckus in the hospital because of their high-handed handling of patients. Why were these faces of managers and corporate businessmen not placed before me in my education?

Why was I not shown videos of the media shouting and calling doctor's looters, murderers, and corrupt? Why were we not told that whatever you do in real life, the sin of a few rotten apples in the profession will bring bad fame to all doctors? Media management is an important topic in the world, and why was that left off my curriculum? When these people want treatment, they will always go to big hospitals and get free treatment in the name of the media, but when it comes to showing the real truth of any story related to doctors, they will start with doctors as the culprits.

Violence against doctors has become common in India. Somedays I feel we will require boxers to protect us like big businessmen. Why were lessons on self-defense not in my curriculum? Just a few months ago, a lady doctor was hacked to death by relatives. A doctor was beaten so badly that he lost his eyes; another lost his hearing; and someone lost his hand. If I fail, they beat me; if I don't answer as per their liking, they beat me; if some managers delay their treatment or overcharge them, they beat me; if the government doesn't clarify about the insurance program started by them, they beat me. Why we were not imparted a self-defense lesson during our curriculum?

When we were studying, we heard from our parents that there are LIC, Mediclaim, and term policies. We never knew that apart from relatives, someone without any medical knowledge and without being directly present at the scene of treatment would ask me why I have admitted this patient, why I have kept this patient for extra days, and why this treatment was given, and so on. We will not pay for treatment and consultation for diabetes, heart disease, or kidney disease as this is a surgical patient. Why were insurance companies and their tricks of not paying clients not taught to us?

This book will show all this as it happened during my to-date practice of medicine. I guess many more things are yet to come.

When will we doctors finally be laid to rest in peace or allowed to practice in peace?

Contents

Maybe Some Of You May Understand And Relate- An Introduction   1

Do What Is Right. Stand Up For Your Colleague.   3

A Fatal Mistake, A Life Lost A Future Lesson Learned   9

The System Is There To Make Your Life Complicated. More If You Are Part Of The System   15

Life Is Lost, But Politics Is Important. And Politics Likes To Have Scapegoat   24

Your Treatment Saves Lives, But Your Paperwork Saves You.   30

All Were Happy, But What About The Donkey?   35

You Are My Competitors, So Remain An Average Doctor. Absurd And Shameful   40

I Am Also Human But Still A Doctor. Empathy And Care Are A Must.   47

Own The Responsibility. Respect The Colleague. Otherwise, There Is No Respect.   52

Nothing Is Better Than Nature, The Finest Teacher And The Finest University On Earth.   56

Doctor, Do You Have A Family? You Seem To Be On Duty All The Time.   63

Humans Are The Worst Enemies Of Humans. No One Can Challenge This.   69

Lots Of Suffering And Lots Of Learning—A Better Doctor In Making   74

Politics And Religion Are Winners, But Humanity Is A Big Loser. For Doctors, Later Is Important.   77

Time To Get The Final Degree. Hurray   82

Oh Man. This Was Not In The Book. And This Is Just The Start   86

The Hospital Is Not The Only Educator; The Family Is Also. The Real Face Of Corporate Doctors   94

Come On, People, Stand Up And Welcome Dr. Gupta .Will He Be Part Of The Rat Race? Only Time Will Tell.   100

A Jolt And Loss Of Money, But Lessons Learnt Helped To Survive. 103

It's Time To Do A Solo Practice. I Am Self-Employed Now, But I Am A Daily Wager. 114

Hypocrisy Of The Highest Nature—But Some Doctors Are Known For That. 118

Managers Will Be Managers. A Life Lost And A Lesson Learned. 122

Without Good Friends, Life Is Depressing. In This Medical Profession They Keep You Sane. 132

We Doctors Are Criminals For The Larger Society. But Why? 144

I Never Thought About Such Changes In Corporate Culture. This Is A Definite Self-Destruction Mode. 148

The Era Of Migration With A Dream Of Better Managers And Work Cultures. 155

Policymakers Have No Knowledge About Medical Practice. They Only Know How To Order. 157

The Future Of Healthcare In India That I See 162

About The Author 165

Maybe Some Of You May Understand And Relate - An Introduction

Doctors in any part of the world don't become what they are because of the books they study. Books and professors teach them the human body. But dealing with humans and learning from them happens as they age and as they grow. Some become compassionate, some are rude and practical, and some are very professional.

The culture where one is born, the family where your upbringing happens in earlier years, the lifestyle one has lived in the early days, and the one that he or she has dreamed of at a later stage shape one's mind. With that mind, dealing with multiple different humans during practice makes the final entity a different species called "Doctor".

I was born into a middle-class family that has given importance to education for the last four generations. Be it a boy or a girl, education was important before entering into anything else. So from early standards, my whole aim was to get good merits in school.

My parents were a middle-class couple with lots of members in a joint family. My father in particular took pride in spending everything he earned on brothers and sisters and their kids. In that process, he completely forgot that he himself had two kids. So from childhood, I knew I could survive with less money and basic amenities. Luxury, outings, vehicles, and trips were not on my bucket list from childhood.

I lived in a joint family. When I was 7 years old, the age where you understand lots of things, I had five generations living under the same roof. Right from my great-great-grandfather to me, there was a whole range of age groups in the family. So basically, I could see all the gametes of disease in the family itself. The routine of going to the doctor and having lots of reports, medicines, operations, and admissions was familiar to me from childhood. So basically, I could see what havoc it can have on a middle-class family. One sick person in the family meant the whole family's finances went berserk. And in that case, if the family doctor advised more reports or referred to a higher center or super specialty, then the next few months could be very difficult for even a nuclear family. So getting sick was not allowed until one had no strength to suffer more.

So with this background, I finally entered a medical course. My bookish education gave me the degree to practice medicine with authority. I had a degree and a license to practice, which was enough to enter the game. But was that the case? Let's see.

During my MBBS days, it was all about the rat race. Books and books, lectures after lectures—it was just cramping. Marks and merits were all that counted. If you could answer tricky questions and out-of-the-box questions, you were considered a genius. The results of the exam put you in the category of geniust. But that's how it is. So after five and a half years of study, I got my MBBS degree. But I guess that gave me the prefix Doctor and nothing else. I had no confidence in seeing a single patient. Through this whole five and a half years, the only thing I knew was individual disease. What are the ideal symptoms for investigation and medicine? But humans don't present themselves like books. So the degree gave me the ego of being a doctor but also made me learn my first lesson. It taught me that this is not enough. In fact, with this book's language, I could easily kill more people than save them. I could easily hurt more people than help them. So I guess it was an indication that I need to study more. And since I liked medicine, I took a 3 years of Internal medicine course to become a physician. In these 3 years, the main methodology is working as a doctor on duty in government hospitals under professors. We are supposed to run the OPD, see patients, and treat them on a regular basis. If admitted, then we need to treat them accordingly and give rounds twice daily to the professors, who subsequently help us finalize the therapy. In an emergency, we need to attend to critical patients and provide standard care to save their lives. This may appear simple to many, but believe me, this is the most stressful life that a young mind lives while working to safeguard the lives of so many patients with whatever limited knowledge he or she knows. But this learning curve makes us complete doctors who, in later stages, can independently treat and manage any patient in their specialty.

How we doctors become what we are is through these phases. Every patient can teach us to become better, more professional, and more expert doctors. But one thing is also true these same things make us learn things that are not written in books.

Do What Is Right. Stand Up For Your Colleague.

When I joined my medical unit at VS Hospital in Ahmedabad, I got the shock of my life. In any unit, there are three types of students. First-year students are there to carry out all the orders of the senior students and the professors. All the paperwork is their job. The first year is supposed to see the patient, write all the history, fill out all forms, draw the blood if needed, write the treatment, make sure that all this blood reaches the laboratory, take patients for x-rays or sonographies, properly give medicines, and attend any emergencies that come up with the admitted patients. All this is done under the guidance of second- or third-year students. So in short, a first-year student is like a clerk doing all the heavy lifting for the unit. Without him, day-to-day work in a government hospital can come to a standstill. But when I joined my unit, I found that I had no second or third year to help me. So basically, I was given the duty to be all three years from day one.

Wednesday was an emergency and OPD day for my medical unit 3. I entered Ward 1 on the ground floor. It was a male patient ward for medical units 1, 2, and 3. As I entered, the ward was full of patients, and there was a huge commotion inside the ward. There were three rows of patients. One row of 10 patients was from unit 1, another middle row of 10 was from unit 2, and the last 10 patient rows were from unit 3.

Tuesday was Emergency Day and Opd Day in Medical Unit 2, where the first year like me was Dr. Dalal. He has been a good friend of mine since my MBBS days. As such, all six unit doctors in the first year were from the same batch of 1994 and have been together in MBBS studies for five and half years. So it was a good environment in the wards, as we complimented each other well. Except for a few who consider themselves privileged, rest of us were good friends.

The commotion was routine in the morning. Every day, my morning ward would be full because of the previous day's emergency. Since units 1, 2, and 3 were allotted to ward 1, the ward remained chockablock until Thursday morning. So Dr.Dalal had a bad emergency day. He almost had

45 admissions throughout the 24-hour emergency day. He could not sleep for a second and also missed both meals.

Wednesday was my emergency day. As such, on a day of emergency, the morning is light as most of the patients from the previous emergency day are discharged and hardly 4 to 5 patients are left admitted. So in the morning, Dr. Dalal was in a mess, and I was a bit relaxed. Dr. Dalal has not yet gone to his room to take a bath. This is the routine for all first-year students on days of emergencies and days after that. We both have made it a habit, along with Dr. V.D (a first-year colleague of Medical Unit 5) in these initial days, to help each other. We did this with two intentions first, this could lighten each other's work, and second, we could see more patients this way.

Senior sister Madhuben was shouting at Dr. Dalal, "Doctor, be fast. Still, five patients are left without a vein. You have been in this ward for a month, and still you have not gained speed in taking veins. If you don't do it before the round starts, then I will not give any injections till 2 p.m".

I shouted, "But sister, your junior sisters are sitting in the room chatting and laughing. Why don't you send them to help Dr. Dalal? Is it not the work of staff to take veins and give medicines".

Sister Kalpana "Oh ho. See how much pain he is in? Dr. Gupta, don't act smart. Remember, today is your emergency. We will make sure that no work is done for your patients. Let's see how your boss reacts in the morning when patients and relatives will be shouting."

Sister Madhu "Listen, all you first years. Remember, don't try to teach us our work. Silently do all the work. When you admit a patient from the OPD to the ward, make sure all forms are properly filled out. Otherwise, that patient will be left till last."

Dr. Sharda, though she was junior to Miss Madhu and Miss Kalpana, was the shrewdest of all. Every staff member and even many of the bosses feared her. She could stall all the work, she could create chaos in the hospital, and she could even start a strike. She was part of the nursing union.

She entered the conversation "It looks like we have a batch who like to care for fellow doctors. So let's do one thing. Let them work for each other and help each other. Why don't Dr. Gupta and Dr. Dr. Dalal take the veins of the remaining patients and give all the injections? Both of you do the same thing in each other's emergencies. Our staff will not work for your units."

I shouted angrily. Since it was only the first month and since I have been running around all wards, emergency rooms, and OPD since day one, I thought this senior staff would sympathize and help. But instead, she was trying to make life hell for me. Because of this, I could never go back to my room, even for meals.

"Sister, this is pure absurdity. How can you do so? We are all working for patients, and each of us has some responsibilities. Because of this absurd order of yours, me and Dr. Dr. Dalal will definitely suffer, but patients will be the ultimate sufferers. Please understand this".

Sister Sharda "Oh, now you remember patients. Doctor, you are working here for patients and for your degree. We are doing our job and will get our salaries anyhow. So don't teach us moral lessons. Now move on. Remember, in half an hour, both your bosses will be here for rounds."

Miss Sharda "And believe me, I will make sure this order is not only for ward 1 but for ward 10, the Jain ward, and the emergency room as well." Now let's see how you survive this. Now go play Bhai Bhai."

I was very angry. And I decided to take this matter to my sir. I then remembered something. Sister Sharda, why have you punished only me and Dr. Dalal? Why is this not applicable to Dr. Desai and Dr. Vats?"

Miss Sharda " You are not the one to decide about this. These two doctors are doing their jobs well. Their boss is the superintendent of this hospital. Also, these two people bring pens, a diary, a keychain, and many more gifts that MR gives in OPD. Dr. Vats, in fact, has become our friend. She brings teas and snacks in the evening for all of us. So we will also play friend friend.

I saw both our colleagues in unit I. They were both smiling cunningly. Though they were part of our team for five and a half years, they were always opportunistic. They never came to help any of us, though they would be free. Instead, they would boast about the teaching they got from their seniors and how they got time to study books.

Books in the first year after graduation were unheard of. But their unit head was the superintendent of the hospital. So they had two doctors every year. So they had doctors on duty for each ward. Life teaches so much.

My anger increased. Since it was a matter of morning rounds, which could get embarrassing if work is not finished before the professors come for a round, we both decided to hurry. We both worked like slaves for the next 45 minutes. We took veins from almost 12 patients and gave them all the injections as written in the order. Both of us finished writing the day's fresh orders in the case paper with all the findings. The handwriting was normally so bad, and it got worse that day. We both can't read what we have written. One of us ran to the laboratory to collect the reports of all the patients. One ran towards the radiology department to get all the appointments for the patients. As we came back to the ward, we both were perspiring like in an oven. Still, we continued our work. All the reports were kept in the case papers, and just as we were doing our last work, Dr. Dr. Dalal saw his head of the unit, Dr. U.Shah, entering the ward. He skipped his heartbeat. He knew today that he was completely in a mess.

As Dr. Shah entered the ward, Sharda sister suddenly came and started talking to him. She was actually speaking loudly, so we could all listen to her. "Sir, it looks like your new resident doctor likes to complain more and do less work. He, along with Dr. Gupta, are constantly reminding us about our job and responsibilities. I don't think they can survive the first year.

Dr.Shah gave an angry look to Dr. Dalal. Though he was looking angrily at Dr. Dalal, I felt a shiver down my spine. I knew this was going to create more problems for Dr. Dalal.

My anger was now replaced by the thought of my head of the unit responding similarly to a complaint by the sister.

I saw Dr. Dalal being thrashed verbally at every patient by Dr. U. Shah. He shouted at Dr. Dalal from every bed. What made it even worse was not that the head of the unit was shouting, but that the patient on that bed and the relatives around him were also looking at Dr. Dalal as someone who knew nothing. So now, after the round, all the patients and relatives will disrespect Dr. Dalal and treat him like some culprit.

Dr. Dalal looked very depressed. He had been awake for the last 26 hours, had not taken food, and was in a mess. With this incident, the coming 5 to 6 days will also be worse.

As I saw my head of unit, Dr. Modi, enter the ward, my heartbeat raced like a Formula One car. And then, out of the corner of my eyes, I saw the same sister approaching him at a rapid pace.

I thought of running away from the ward, never to be found. But then that would be the end of my career, even before it started. So I slowly moved towards the group. The sister was explaining something to my professor. Then, with a wicked smile, she stepped aside and moved towards the desk.

As my boss saw me, he came towards me and, with a wink, asked me, "Looks like your residency has started. You should have really messed with Sister's ego". Laughingly, he continued, Don't bother; keep doing your work. We all know how stressed you are because of the absence of any residents with you. Don't let her bother you".

I felt a cool breeze of air on my head. It was like a dream. I realized then what it meant to be the head of a unit. Sir has seen almost 30 residents in his long career; he has been in this hospital for the last 30 years, and he has known this staff since then. So basically, he knew what they were capable of.

My round went as planned. My boss was a very clinical doctor. Nothing missed his eyes. He asked all the relevant questions and gave relevant advice. His teaching was also a mix of education and a practical approach. He always said to every resident **"What you study is for passing the exam. Books are for exams. But in practice, things are different. You deal with real life, and only experience matters."**

But after this episode, my relationship with a group of nursing staff worsened. Sharda sister and gang made it their aim to harass me and Dr. Dalal almost at every instance. They would not take any veins from patients, delay the medicine in patients, and many a day would make a few of the reports vanish. The fight between me and this gang escalated at every level. I was not ready to take things lying down. For me, it affected my routine and often put the lives of patients in danger.

But another thing happened because of that. A lot of other staff who had also been working here for 30 to 35 years started respecting us. They saw intent in our things. They saw how we rushed to help every patient.

Dr. Dalal and I were always present in case of need among our fellow residents. This also made our faces visible in the hospital. We did this as we got more exposure to patients from different units. We were present in rounds with other units in the evening. In the evening, it was a protocol where the senior resident of the unit used to take rounds. They used to see whether all things were done properly or not; reports were collected; medicines were proper. This helped them be ready for the professor's round in the morning. Also, this helps juniors learn and correct anything wrong with the patients. But in my unit, I was alone. So I never had any rounds or suggestions from any senior, right from the beginning. My second year was sent on rotation in different specialties like neurology, cardiology, nephrology, and gastroenterology. My third year was most cunning, and so he came directly for morning rounds. He was my professor's favorite resident. So being present in other unit rounds in the evening helped me learn faster, and I also got suggestions from the seniors in those units for my complicated patients.

While we were becoming doctors, our learning came in many forms. Day to day, we learned by watching our seniors and professors treat the patients. How they took the history and what is important in the history helps to decide the next step. Then clinical examinations and their interpretations, then the reports advised, and finally the treatment given either with surety or with a hunch The response that we see in the patient gives us insight about the whole process. Along with this, we learn how our seniors and professors are interacting and communicating with the patient and their relatives. This communication was also the most important tool for giving proper treatments.

Apart from these day-to-day uncommon events that happen in hospitals, they also help us understand the uncertainty of the process.

One wrong thing can take someone's life. A rigid patient or relative can make suffering worse.

A Fatal Mistake, A Life Lost A Future Lesson Learned

It was Friday morning. Unit 5 was getting ready for long hours ahead as it was their emergency. Unit 4 residents were rushing everywhere to be ready for rounds after long emergency hours. Rest units were a bit relaxed as their period of long hours was over for this week.

But around 9.15 am, suddenly there was chaos all around in Ward 2. Here were patients from Units 4, 5, and 6. As I mentioned earlier, there were three rows of patients in each unit.

Suddenly, two patients in units 4 and 6 worsened together. On one side of the row at the end, near the wall, was Bhikhabhai of Unit 4. Dr. Bhagat, my fellow first-year resident of Unit 4, suddenly rushed towards his patient.Bhikhabhai was gasping for air, and his body was cold. He could not speak.

Bhikhabhai "please do something". He could not even finish these words properly. His relatives were shouting for help.

Bhagat"Sister, please bring the oxygen bottle here. Please get me the blood pressure instrument."

Dr.Bhagat to the relatives ' Looks like Bhikhabhai has worsening heart failure". He came in with heart failure and was recovering. He was in the ICU for three days, where he fought death valiantly and was winning with the help of doctors.

Dr. Bhagat" Sister, what happened? He was looking good when I took rounds just half an hour ago. His parameters looked good then."

He kept shouting, "Sister, come fast. Bring an injection of Lasix and give it early."

He shouted at the ward boy, "Brother. Run fast and bring a stretcher. We need to shift him to the ICU. Don't walk like a tortoise."

He was frantically doing all that he knew. He was in this clinical practice for only one month. So his knowledge of how to treat a seriously ill patient was limited. But still, he was trying everything he knew. Luckily, he got the help of a senior resident, Dr. Ruchir from Unit 2, who was there for his rounds in Ward 1.

Dr. Ruchir of Unit 2 shouted the moment he saw the patient. ``This is bad pulmonary edema. The patient's heart and lung have failed, and so he is having pink, frothy sputum. He is going to go into cardiac arrest."

He asked the sister, "What were the morning medicines that were given to this patient?"

The junior sister picked up her nursing book to see the medicine given to each patient by her.

She said, "I have given her Injection Rantac, an antibiotic injection, and an Inject Atropine 6 ampoule."

There was pin-drop silence among the doctors standing around. Dr. Bhagat had beads of perspiration on his face.

Dr. Bhagat angrily shouted, " Holy sh*t!" He was so angry that he shouted many curse words loudly. Though embarrassing, he could not help. "Don't you know this patient is suffering from heart failure? His ejection fraction on admission was hardly 20 percent. It took us five days to stabilize him. And how can you give him injection. Atropine?"

When this commotion was going on, exactly on the opposite side, relatives of a patient in Unit 6 started shouting."Doctor, sister, please come here. My husband is not opening his eyes; he is breathing so fast. Please save him".

Now it was the turn of Dr. Ritesh to run. He shouted, Sister, bring an oxygen saturation machine and a blood pressure instrument. Start oxygen in him.Since he had already heard about the medicines given to the patient by Dr. Bhagat, he was sure what had happened.

His patient had organophosphorus poisoning. Atropine is a life-saving injection given as an antidote to save such patients. But this injection leads to a rise in pulse to 150 above, makes the patient violent, and makes him dry.

He shouted, "Where is the senior staff? He asked the junior staff, "Rush and bring injection atropine 6 ampoule and give it to this patient. And arrange for him to be shifted to the ICU immediately".

By this time, the patient of Dr. Bhagat had suffered cardiac arrest. He and the senior resident, Dr. Ruchir, were giving cardiac massage to the patient.

These were the days when no facility was available in wards to intubate the patient to put him on a ventilator. There was no Crash Cart, which had all emergency medicine. In about 15 minutes, frantic chest compressions gave no result. Finally, Dr. Ruchir declared the patient dead. The relatives cried loudly and were inconsolable. They were very angry, and one of them started banging on the table and was about to get violent. But by then, the ward boys had come and taken him out of the ward. They consoled him and kept him in check.

Dr. Ruchir was now very disturbed, but his rounds had started in Ward 1. So he hurriedly went to his ward.

Senior staff did come, but instead of scolding the junior sister for such grave mistakes, she shouted at Dr. Bhagat. "You first-year residents are so careless. You knew the patient was serious, so why did you bring him to the ward? Why were you not with the staff to give injections? My junior sister cannot understand this big medical term of heart failure and pulmonary edema. See, your carelessness has killed the patient."

Dr. Bhagat was like lava inside, about to burst. He lost all his control "How dare you say this to me? What are you sisters here for? You come here and gossip. You spend the whole day cutting vegetables and talking bullshit. These sisters and you are good for nothing. Instead of accepting your mistakes, you are blaming me. I have clearly written the orders of medicine with timing."

By then, the head of the unit, Dr.Mehta, had arrived. He silenced all of them and asked them to come to the doctor's console, a separate room for doctors and staff.

Dr. Mehta "Dr. Bhagat, don't shout like this in front of patient relatives. They have just lost their patient, and hearing you like this can cause more trouble".

Dr. Bhagat "But sir, this sister is blaming me and saying I killed the patient. The junior sister was the one who gave injection atropine to the patient, which caused heart failure and pulmonary edema, which led to cardiac arrest".

Dr. Mehta "Sister, is this true?"

Senior staff "Sir, I agree that injection atropine was given to the patient by my staff. But how can they know that this is a heart failure patient? And above this, all the residents of three units keep their case papers here and there. In the morning, you also know how chaotic it is. We are taking all parameters, like temperature and all; we are giving sponges to sick patients; and we are writing all the notes in our charts. Beside this, we are rushing to do all the work of the previous day's emergency patients."

Dr. Mehta "I can understand this. But it was your sister who gave the wrong injection. Then why blame the residents? You are insulting him and also breaking his morals."

Senior staff has now lost all respect for the professor as well. She rudely said, "See, Dr. Mehta, control your residents. Don't teach us what is right and wrong. Don't tell us we are to blame. Otherwise, I will inform our nursing union, and we will then see what happens."

Dr. Mehta was very angry, but with his experience of 30 years in this government hospital, he knew what would happen once the nursing union came into play.

He silently moved out of the room and asked Dr.Bhagat to follow. They went and met the relatives and tried to pacify them. After that, the round of Unit 4 was very depressing and silent.

In the evening, we all make it a point to meet in the hostel and discuss our day-to-day work. This became a routine for all eight of us. There were 6 units, but units 1 and 4 had 2 first-year residents each, and the rest had one. As such, the whole day, be it ward, opd, lunch time, or evening ward, the topic of discussion was the death of the patient. The lives of the resident doctors are such that time for introspection is too short. Patients in OPD, new or old, admissions, emergencies, rounds, politics of nursing staff, politics of senior residents, collection of reports, meticulously writing case papers, and health literacy of patients took all the time. In fact, 24 hours appeared to be a very short day.

The death was to be discussed when there was leisure time. So come evening, when seven of us sat in the hostel (the eighth one was absent as it was his emergency), the topic was the death of the patient.

Dr. Bhagat "It is so absurd. A patient dies because of the fault of that sister, but the blame is on us. The senior staff even threatened to go to the union and create chaos".

Dr. Dalal "Leave it, Bhagat. We should learn from this. Let's be cautious from now on."

Dr. Desai Yes, Dr. Dalal is right. If we know that a patient is serious and has recovered after a critical illness, then we need to be proactive. In our unit, our professor has said, on day 1, check all the medicines."

Bhagat "Don't be stupid. Checking medicine is done in our unit as well. But then, do you give injections to patients in your unit? No na. Then stop acting and understand. This patient died because that staff gave an injection that was to be given to the patient of Dr. Ritesh."

Ritesh "Yes. Bhagat is right. Atropine given to a heart failure patient is gross negligence. But it is the staff who are responsible. If Bhagat had written atropine in his order, then only it was his fault."

Bhagat and Ritesh are right practically. But even if it is the fault of staff, ward boys, or hospital services, the blame is first put on doctors".

Dr. Vats Like the USA, soon for every wrong, first a doctor will be blamed. By then the media will be powerful, laws will be misused, lawyers will be there to win, and we doctors will have a hell of a ride".

Bhagat " I don't care what happens after 10 years. As of now, I am sure we are all going to learn more about the system along with how to treat the patient."

We are to blame in healthcare for everything that goes wrong. But let's be vigilant. Remember, this is a general hospital. Patients are really poor and needy. And above all, have no health literacy. So let's work together and be careful."

Ritesh "I am not sure if Lasix was given to my patient instead of Dr. Bhagat's patient. Mine has been passing urine in tons since morning."

Though it was tragic and one patient did lose their life, we laughed. That's another change that has happened to us since the day we joined residency.

Dr Vora" Since MBBS, this is the most dangerous change that has happened to all of us."

What is that, Dr. Vora?"

She said, "We have thick skin."

I laughed. "Ya, you are right. Seeing our professors, staff, and other paramedics moving around doing their routine life things with ease even with so much suffering has made us also the same."

Bhagat" Yes, today only after the death of the patient, staff were enjoying their tea and snacks with gossip and loud laughter. The relatives were crying outside around the bed of the patient who died, and here they were shouting, laughing, and boasting as to how Dr. Mehta could not say a thing to senior staff.

Dr.Dalal "Daily we see this. So I guess that's how it is."

Ritesh "Why aren't just staff, even our seniors, our professors are used to all this? They say if you stop your routine life after seeing someone suffer, then you cannot become a doctor. We doctors, and in fact the whole healthcare system, have to realize that if we want to help patients, we need to be practical and professional."

Dr Vora "Yeah, they are right as such. But really, it is difficult to do that immediately. I have nightmares many nights. I see my patient screaming."

Dr. Dalal "Just a few days ago, I saw Sister Sharda laughing loudly in my dreams. I got up with perspiration and rapid heartbeats."

We all laughed. We all knew about the episode of Dr. Dalal and me with Sister Sharda.

Dr Vora "So it appears our ego of getting into postgraduate MD internal medicine has already crashed. We will be doctors, but we will be heavily dependent on so many people."

Dr Desai"So right. As physicians, we will be dependent on patients telling us the right history. Then pathology to give proper reports. Then pharmaceutical companies to give quality, proper medicines, and then again, patiently follow things meticulously."

I said "So right. But I guess we will do well. If we learn properly and take proper care while treating. And if we communicate well, I guess we will do fairly well".

The System Is There To Make Your Life Complicated. More If You Are Part Of The System

In our hospital, there were some rules regarding OPD and admissions. We have professors who were allowed to practice in private. So they had their OPDs outside also. Every patient was recognized as a new patient (who had come to the hospital for the first time) and an old patient. In older patients, if the patient comes to the hospital other than their unit days in an emergency, they will be admitted to the emergency medical unit.

The next day, this patient would be transferred to the parent unit (every patient's OPD book has the parent unit name written). But if any patient came and got admitted with the private prescription of the professor, then the book was not considered, but that prescription became important. Then that patient became a patient of the professor's unit.

I had two professors. One was head of unit Dr. Modi, and another was associate professor Dr. DAM. Both had their clinics outside. So like other units, we also got transfers every now and then from other units if there was an old patient who got admitted to the emergency unit or if my professors had sent their patient to the emergency unit.

It was Friday morning. I got a transfer case from Unit 4, which had an emergency on Thursday. Getting new patients like this always irritates first-year residents. So first, we always try to find out if there are any mistakes in the papers. So I did the same, and I got one. Elated, I shouted at Bhagat.

Dr. Bhagat, "Why are you giving this transfer to us? She has an old OPD book for Unit 1. Our superintendent has been seeing her for the last year. Transfer her to unit 1".

Dr. Mukesh sir was our superintendent as well as head of the department of medicine. He was head of Unit 1. He had an air of arrogance, because of which many of the professors did not like him.

Bhagat, laughingly "Sorry, Gupta, bad luck. But as you know, this patient, Mrs. Shah, is senior staff in Ward 2. And though she was a regular patient of our superintendent, she has consulted your professor in private and brought his prescription for admission. So as per rule, she has to be transferred under your unit."

I shouted at the patient, "Why didn't you show me the prescription, sir? You are unnecessarily creating chaos here. You are senior staff, and don't you know the rules?"

Mrs. Shah" Dr. Lower your voice. Stop shouting and do your work."

I got irritated, but I knew it would not help. So I started asking about the clinical history.

"So tell me, what are your complaints?"

Mrs. Shah " I have had an on-and-off fever for 1 year. It comes every 20 to 25 days and lasts for 5 to 6 days. I also have a bodyache and headache."

"Do you have chills, a cough, diarrhea, or abdominal pain?" I was rushing for questions.

Mrs. Shah "Doctor, it appears you are least bothered about history. You are doing this as a formality."

Sister, "Why don't you answer the questions and stop passing judgments? You should know that Dr. Modi will be here soon. Then I will have time only until 3 p.m. Do you want to suffer till then"?

Mrs. Shah knew I was all alone in the unit. So my rounds will be long, and then after each round, work will take a lot of time. I have been going for my lunch almost every day at around 3 p.m. because of this. By this time, all my colleagues were fast asleep.

Mrs. Shah" In a few of the episodes, I did have chills. One time around, I also had diarrhea."

"Did you have a cough, cold, or breathing issues?"

She said, "No, doctor, there were no such things".

"Did you have a loss of appetite, bodyache, weakness, easy fatigue, or weight loss?"

She said, "Yes, doctor, all the symptoms are there. In fact, they have increased since last month. I have lost 20 kg or so of weight in the last 6 months."

I asked, "Do you have diabetes or any other illness?"

She said, "No, doctor, I have been investigated many times. I have been admitted as many as 10 to 12 times. I was investigated and treated for malaria, typhoid, and tuberculosis. But every time reports are negative, Dr. Mukesh gives medicine, suspecting all of these."

"Oh, so clinically, you are actually a case of fever of unknown origin. Do you have all the files?"

She said it angrily. "My husband has torn down all the files of Dr. Mukesh. He got angry this time. He said your doctor doesn't know anything. He can't diagnose a simple fever. He has done so many reports, and still he does not know anything."

But, sister, you also know how this type of fever is. A lot of investigations are required, and it is quite possible that all reports can come back normal".

After examining her and reviewing her old files, I wrote down all the relevant points in the case paper. Then I saw all the reports done by my professors. All the reports that he has suggested were done the previous day, and they were all normal. As I was doing my rounds in different units daily, I was learning many things. So I, without asking my professor, sent many other reports.

The routine rounds happened. And after finishing my rounds, I went to my hostel room and slept for a while. Since today was quite an easy day with a lesser number of patients, I got a rare afternoon to sleep. By that time, senior staff member Mrs. Shah had been shifted from the general ward to the special room. Since she was a senior staff member, she got this facility as per the rules.

Around 5 p.m., when I went for my evening rounds, I thought of going to see Mrs.Shah first. The moment I entered the ward, the staff over there rushed toward me and shouted. "What is this Gupta? You have admitted an HIV patient in my ward." I was shell-shocked.

"What nonsense. I have only one patient in your ward. That is your own colleague, Mrs. Shah. So you are mistaken. Go find the right doctor to blame and shout."

Then I got the shock of life." Doctor, I am talking about your patient only. She is HIV positive patient".

"But I have no information about that. How the hell do you know that?"

Then the actual bomb burst" The pathology lab has sent an envelope in the name of Mrs. Shah. So I took it and read it. And she says she is positive."

I shouted, "You are senior staff here. You should know that the envelope is a sealed cover, and that should only be given to the doctor of the unit. He or she can only open it and do what is needed. You know this will lead to a break in the privacy cycle of the patient."

She angrily said, "You stop teaching me protocols. It was a report from our colleague. So out of curiosity, I opened it. And you are blaming me."

By this time, I had learned that there was no point fighting with full-time staff, ward boys, and other staff of the hospital. They have their own way of functioning, and they were all part of one or another union. So I gave up.

Sister, "So how many people know about this except me?"

She said, "Don't act smart. I am not a news channel. I have not told anyone. After opening the envelope, I went to our cafeteria. There were only senior staff, and so I have mentioned these to them. Don't worry, only the sister in charge of ward 1, ward 2, ward 10, and Jain ward knows about this."

I almost thought of banging her head with the hammer that I had for the neurology examination. But better sense prevailed, and I asked for the envelope.

" I hope you have not told that to the patient and her relatives."

She saw me through the corner of her eyes" Do you think I am a fool? No, I have not told her. It's just that when I was talking to a Jain ward sister, her son heard it. But then he is just a 10-year-old kid. Don't worry, he will not know what HIV positive means".

I was actually very angry inside, boiling like lava, but my past experience has taught me that no one will stand with me in this matter either.

I"Ok, sister. Thanks for all the help."

I then went straight to the telephone operator near the emergency ward. Since the only telephone available to make a public call was near the emergency ward, every resident had to go there to talk to their professors.

I called Dr. DAM and informed him about the report. He was shell-shocked" But I never advised the HIV report. Who got it done?"

I thought he was angry and would blast me. I bluntly told the lie "Sir, she was with unit 4 yesterday, so maybe they sent it."

Dr. DAM" How dare they send anything apart from what I have advised in my prescription? Who are they to interfere in my management?"

That day, I learned a new lesson. Whoever sent the report, it was this report that finally gave a name to the disease of the senior staff. She has been on treatment for a year without a diagnosis and has not found any relief. Today, with this report, we can stamp that her fever was caused by HIV. Now at least we know which road we need to go on, and even relatives will get an answer. But instead of thanking the resident who sent the report, my professor was having an ego spell. **It appears that the doctor community has a huge ego in which they may become blind many times.**

Now it was my professor's turn to panic. Sir "Gupta, today read about the HIV and management part briefly. We will have an update lecture tomorrow. It is a nice case of fever of unknown origin".

I was like, "What the hell? I cannot read now. I don't get time to eat, and my professor wants me to study a topic that requires months to finish."

My soul was shouting, One hundred percent he himself wants to learn about further investigation and treatment plans.

I asked him, Sir, what should I do next?" Should I tell the patient or relatives? What further investigation should I send? What medicine should I start?"

Before my list of queries kept rising, he shouted, "Gupta, stop. Don't tell her or her relatives. No new meds, only symptomatic medicine. We need to confirm this and also see her status in terms of disease and severity. Till then, just take a routine round.

I was a bit relieved by this order. Now I don't need to give exams to patients or relatives. At least I will have the rest of the day in peace. Later tomorrow, let my professor face the music of interrogation.

Remember, it was 1999–2000. This disease, though seen frequently, had a huge stigma.

Dr. Bhatt was the senior resident of Unit 5. He met me in routine rounds, and so after he completed taking rounds with Dr. Dr. V.D, I caught him and started asking him about the disease.

"Sir, what should be my next step"?

He was irritated but still calm. He knew my condition. "Gupta, first send the confirmatory reports of Western Blot, and then once you get that report, send the CD4 count to decide the stage. Apart from this, let your professor decide about the therapy, as there are multiple regimens, and also about other infections that we call opportunistic infections ".

Though I have read about this disease in MBBS, now that I was actually dealing with it in a real scenario, things went like a bouncer to me. Already, I was burdened by so much work, and on top of that,

Still, I have to do what is to be done. So I went back to the ward of that patient and ordered a Western blot. Then I got another shock.

Senior Staff "Doctor, where should we keep this patient? She cannot be in our ward. This is a VIP ward, and people here will panic if they come to know that there is an HIV patient here."

I literally shouted, "Sister, what rubbish are you talking about? This is a hospital. Different patients come here. We can't discriminate like this".

"And remember, she is your colleague. Why are you doing this to her?"

She shouted and blurted out the real reason "Doctor, we all have families. Why should I, my staff, ward boy, and sanitation worker risk their health? Would she not infect us?"

I never thought I would hear this" So you mean we also should not give treatment as we also have family? This is so absurd. We are here to help and treat. And who told, you would get infected if you treated her, gave her injections, took blood, or did her to daycare?"

Sister" You are doing this because you want a degree, and then you can earn a lot as a doctor. We are here for life with so little salary. So don't equate you with us. And I don't know all this. Just shift her."

I also shouted, "No, this is the wrong attitude. You know that this disease is not contagious, and it can come to us only if body fluids are transferred to us. If you do this, then future generations of staff will also engage in this inhuman behavior."

Sister has now lost all sense of decency. "Doctor, don't act smart. Don't teach your bookish language. As I said, just transfer her wherever you want, but away from my ward."

These loud arguments have already drawn a decent crowd. Junior sisters, ward boys, and other helpers were nodding in acceptance of the senior staff's speech. Few of the relatives around were so confused as to what type of disease the patient had that even staff were not ready to take care. They were also getting panicky and fearful.

I knew this would create a huge uproar in a short time. So I cut the argument short and shouted. "Sister, do whatever you wish. Transfer wherever you wish. I have no authority to choose the ward or bed. So talk to the management and do whatever you feel. I don't care. Just inform me of the ward where she is shifted."

I rushed out of the ward after writing the order of the Western blot report.

On the way, I met Dr. Dr. Dalal, and we moved towards our work in the male ward.

"Dr. Dalal, it appears more than the art of clinical work and management, we are also supposed to learn the art of handling relatives, staff, fellow doctors, and so many other things. It is exhausting many times".

Dr. Dalal" The trouble is, patients are so unreliable. They don't tell the right history; they don't know the history many times, and they even don't do what we tell them to do. Illiteracy and poverty, along with corruption, are beyond imagination".

We went on talking about various issues while walking. After reaching the ward, we got into our work.

The evening was like a maze. You see the progress of the patient throughout the day. If any reports are sent, then we collect them and write each thing in the case paper. Then we check the medications that they have to see if all is well or not. Evening times, relatives are also there, and so their questions are there, which we try to answer as per our maturity. Then after that, we write down the orders for the next day on a fresh sheet.

Suddenly, I heard a loud fight between Dr. V.D and her sister. Dr. V.D was very angry as he could not find the patient's case paper. Even the reports were not there that were sent in the morning.

He shouted" You, staff, are taking salary for just coming here, gossiping, cutting vegetables, and harassing the residents. Can't you keep the case paper safe? Who took the case paper last?"

Sister" Doctor, we are not your slaves." We are not your servants who will keep case papers safe. Every case paper is below the patient's mattress. Some relatives might have taken it. And you might also have forgotten it somewhere. You talk more than you do work. We see it all when you are working".

Dr. V.D "What nonsense. Instead of helping me find the case papers and reports, you are alleging and accusing me. You people are actually harrasing us day and night. I will file a written complaint with the superintendent. I can't bear all these things".

I and Dr. Dalal rushed towards him. I and Dr. V.D were roommates. He was the most sincere of all. He was meticulous, studious, and took extreme care of his patients. He liked to do things in a systematic way. Because of that, he always kept everyone around him on their toes.

Just the night before, I suddenly woke up hearing someone whispering in the room. When I opened my eyes, I could see Dr. V.D sitting on the floor on a small mattress and praying to Lord Krishna. He lit a candle and whispered the prayer. I was terrified, as I initially thought he had gone mad. I literally shouted, "Oh boss, why are you doing all this? I got frightened. Why don't you do all this in the morning?"

Dr. V.D" Arey, I just returned from the ward. I wanted to pray for one of my patients. He requires favor from God. We have tried all types of management, but he is not showing any signs of improvement. So I wanted to pray to my Lord Krishna to help him. So you sleep and don't disturb me".

I shouted, "Oh man. What nonsense! You are disturbing me. Instead of that, you are blaming me".

I wanted to have a good sleep as the next day was Wednesday, and it was my turn to remain awake for two days continuously. But this prayer of his has disturbed my sleep, and I know now that two days of mine will be full of vomiting due to a bad migraine. I tried to sleep then, but it took me a long time.

So we all knew in the team of junior residents that Dr. V.D was very sensitive. So when he shouted and said what he said, the next few days would be bad not only for him but also for fellow residents. He will shout and get angry at us now if any of us say anything that he does not like.

Dr. Dalal" Come on, Dr. V.D, we both will help you. Sister at least help us trace the reports of this patient. If you can spare one of your junior staff,

Senior sister shouted back, "No one will come because we have a lot of work. These juniors have so much work, and then they have to give it over to the next shift staff. So go find yourself. And Dr., do file a complaint with your superintendent. Let me also see what he does. But let me tell you what will happen to you."

I and Dr. Dalal saw each other. We knew what was coming. So now it is we three who will have to face the brunt of a boycott by staff. But then, by now, we have started enjoying this. We have gathered strength and will.

"Sister, don't say anything. We know what you are capable of. So don't worry. God sees everything. He knows how to handle you, people. Go and cut your vegetables; otherwise, your family may boycott you."

This irked her more" How dare you".

By that time, a few other senior staff members had come around. They knew that a few of the staff were very harsh on first-year residents just to show their superiority. So directly and indirectly, those few supported junior doctors and helped in every way they could. So they came in between us and sent us three doctors away.

Life Is Lost, But Politics Is Important. And Politics Likes To Have Scapegoat

The next day, as my professor came, the real issue with the senior staff member who was admitted with us started. Her husband was informed of the possible disease and its outcome. He was informed about the reports and treatments planned. Her husband was the union leader, and ironically, he was recently suspended by the superintendent for misbehavior on the job. So the situation became messy. It was the superintendent who treated the staff for one year without any success, and above all, her husband was suspended by the same superintendent. So I guess we were in a sandwich position in this situation. But Dr. DAM has categorically told all of us that we don't talk about those things in front of anyone.

He said, "Dr. Gupta, make sure that our head of unit, Dr. Modi, doesn't take her rounds. Don't discuss or utter anything about past treatment failure in front of anyone, especially the relatives or senior staff of the hospital. We will need the help of the superintendent in getting various reports and getting free medicines for the staff".

I understood the practical issues that my professor was telling me about. So he taught me a new lesson. The **present and future problems should be looked at first, and accordingly, patients should be dealt with. If we keep criticizing the past doctors for their unsuccessful treatment, that will hamper trust and also make relatives upset about the whole process. It is always best to discuss the real medical scenario**.

Dr. DAM "See, in this patient, if you go through the whole file of the last year, Dr. Mukesh has done all that anyone would have done. He, or, let's say, even I, would not have asked for an HIV test, looking at the seniority of the staff and the absence of blood transfusions. I did not ask this time either. It was only because of a junior resident who, by mistake, got this report. So by blaming Dr. Mukesh, we will be putting him in dock. And this will only worsen the whole situation."

I" Ok sir. But there is one more issue, sir. Many staff and ward boys are not ready to take care of her, give injections, or even take blood."

Dr. DAM "Oh, is that so? Quite possible. We may look like a family, but healthcare is a divided lot. But don't worry. I know who will help."

So with that, our round went on. Then we reached Ward No. 10. It was a female ward for all six units. So a huge ward with 70 beds and more than six senior staff members and 10 junior staff members working round the clock So it was a grand ward. Again, the situation in this ward was the same as in the other ward. Talking tough and acting tough. A lot of junior residents feared working in this ward. But one thing was very striking. Almost every third-year resident loved coming to this ward. So the juniors in the initial days looked perplexed. Even our professors felt at ease in this ward.

So when, in our free time, we inquired with our seniors, the reality came out. Every senior staff member in this ward was from a well-to-do family, or at least a middle-class family. They have been in this ward for almost 25 to 30 years and have never been transferred. And they are strict with juniors to make them better doctors. And once they see them doing well in their third year after a nightmarish two years of residency, they feel proud. In the third year, they treat every third-year resident like their kid. They pamper them, bring food for them, celebrate their birthdays, and after evening rounds, gossip with them. So once evening rounds are over, all 3rd year residents, if time permits, sit with on-duty senior staff and have a blast.

Dr. DAM and I reached Ward 10 and finished our round-like routine. Then Dr. DAM approached Sister Nancy. She was a senior staff member, very outspoken, and someone who could make any junior resident cry. She was extremely strict with lots of junior residents and staff. She could know every resident's real nature in a few days. After that, if she finds someone who is lazy or negligent towards patient care, that fellow has to deal with her and her colleagues for a full year.

Dr. DAM" How are you, Nancy, sister? How are your kids? I heard the eldest son is doing well in school. Are you planning to send him to medical school "?

Nancy's sister" I am good, sir. Yes, if he wants to do medical studies, we are OK with that."

Dr. DAM" My unit will need help from you and your colleagues."

Sister" I know what you are asking. We learned about this situation just yesterday. So don't worry; we will plan something. But let me tell you, if your resident shows any laziness or negligence, then I will personally make sure that he does not complete his residency."

A shiver went down my spine. But I knew there would be no problem. I also knew this was an opportunity to enter the good books of all this strict staff in a short time.

Dr. DAM, as if reading my mind, said, "Don't worry, sister. I can assure you about Gupta. Since he is all alone, I initially thought he would run away like many others. But he has done his work properly to date and is also learning fast. He is outspoken like you, so maybe you will like his style of work.``

Sister" Yeah, we all know that. He has had many fights with our staff in wards 1 and 2, as well as in the VIP ward yesterday itself. But we have seen him go through all the units to learn. We have seen him doing work for other fellow residents as well. Still, if he runs away from this patient thinking like those staff, then all this good impression will be wiped off".

I liked what she told me about, but I also understood the warning.

So true to her words, sister Nancy and her troop took care of all things senior staff, Mrs. Shah. They fixed their duties to give her injections and take blood reports. They even sat with her to eat so that she could feel relaxed. Looking at this, I understood that knowing things is one thing, but actually practicing them is what matters. We all read that HIV doesn't spread by touching, eating, or chatting with each other. Also, healthcare, with all extra precautions, should provide all possible care to such patients. But in the actual scenario, doing this matters, and I can see this staff doing it in reality.

The reports of the staff came out positive; tragically, her disease has progressed to end-stage, and despite all treatment efforts, she kept deteriorating and went into shock. She was then shifted to the ICU. Here also, Sister Nancy was of constant help. Mrs. Shah fought a valiant battle, but once she was put on a ventilator, her situation kept deteriorating. Throughout this fight, the most perplexing thing was the attitude of the superintendent. I could see how he reacted to our request to indent the medicine or expensive test. In our hospital, if we need free medicine or free reports, we need to send a request to him in a book called the "Indent Book". This was routine in our hospital, as poor patients were present in large numbers. So every evening from every ward, this book will reach him, and he will judiciously give consent. But in Mrs. Shah's case, he acted differently. He would send unnecessary queries. He would delay the sign with absurd excuses. He would permit only half-quantities. But luckily, here also, Sister Nancy became a savior. Whenever she knew that we were asking for some indentation for Mrs. Shah, she would go herself to the superintendent. The moment he sees Sister Nancy, the superintendent will behave as if a class teacher is present. So we started getting our supplies regularly and on time. After a well-fought battle, Mrs. Shah died one morning of sudden cardiac arrest. I was present there, and many other staff members were there. We tried all that morning to prolong her life but eventually failed. It was quite disturbing to lose her. I finished my paperwork and handed it out to emergency staff. After talking to the aggrieved husband, I went to my room to freshen up so that I could come back for my day's work. I have already informed my professor about the death of the sister. According to his instructions, the paper work was finished.

I would have just reached the gate of the hostel when the warden came running and said, "Dr. Gupta, what happened? It looks like the death of the sister has led to a burst of anger in the husband's mind. He has gone to the superintendent's office and destroyed the whole thing. The nursing matron and nursing union have declared a strike against medical negligence during treatment of staff".

"But I have just met the husband 15 minutes ago." He did not say anything to me. He was crying and asking, "What will happen to his son and daughter? And suddenly this! Unbelievable. And sisters are protesting and alleging negligence!"

I continued" So many staff have refused to provide treatment to the staff. And now this hypocrite is alleging negligence. ``

A few of the residents who were coming from the hospital side said, Dr. Gupta, it looks like things are getting out of hand. There are so many people near the clock tower. Nursing staff, ward boys, and union people are all shouting slogans. I even heard someone shouting Dr. DAM has done negligence".

I could not believe this "How come in a matter of a few minutes so many people have accumulated?"

One of the residents said, "Sir, it is around 8 a.m. So there is a shift change. The night shift is leaving for home, and the morning shift is here. So actually, both shifts have made it a large crowd."

Hearing all this, I was a bit worried now. Crowds have no brains, so they can cause a lot of trouble. But still, I thought it was lucky that I had reached the hostel before the accumulation of the crowd. I went to my room to freshen up and get ready for rounds. I came down to take my breakfast, where again there was discussion of the event only. Almost everyone knew the patient belonged to my unit, and so I was the center of attention. Few of them even sarcastically remarked, "Dr. Gupta, we have never heard such a thing in the last so many years. No one has accused our staff of being negligent. It looks like your unit has really failed in giving proper treatment to the staff. ``

I was in no mood to fight or get angry. I was literally tired because of the exhausting seven days of continuous management of staff. So I just said, "Sir, since you are unaware of the whole event, then please don't pass judgment. If you want to know all about the issue, then we may discuss it when I am free and relaxed. As of now, please don't be judgmental."

This also made me realize the problems with healthcare workers. Without knowing if we are ready to accept the blame for a fellow colleague from the aggrieved relatives and pronounce our own fellow doctor or staff member guilty, how can we find the truth? But today was not the day to teach philosophy. So I ate my breakfast silently, keeping my ears closed. Then I moved towards my ward. There were three police vans on the way, guarding the hospital and also keeping the protester at a safe distance. Seeing me, a few of the staff who recognized me started shouting loudly "Hey doctor, tell your professor we will continue this strike. We will make sure the culprits are punished."

A nursing matron standing nearby shouted back to those protestors, "What absurdity are you taking? Why are you shouting and blaming him and his professor? They are not the real culprits. In fact, they are the people who actually found out what she had, and they gave her proper care until the end. So stop this".

This chaos went on for a few more days. There was a police inquiry over the incident of the superintendent's office wreckage, but Dr. Mukesh did not file any case out of sympathy. There was limited media coverage of the incident, with different colors. We got a summons from the superintendent's office within a week of the death. We were informed that, looking at a high-profile case, there will be an inquiry about the treatment of Mrs. Shah and her death. So we were told to be present at the inquiry commission whenever called. Dr. DAM was angry upon hearing this. So he lost his cool for the first time (that's at least the first time I saw my professor show anger). He said, "Dr. Mukesh, what will be the pointers for inquiry? Will that cover this admission or the whole issue of her illness since last year?

Dr. Mukesh" Dr. DAM I know where you're taking this. Don't act smart. I don't decide the pointers, but they will be decided by the commission. So prepare yourself for the questioning."

Your Treatment Saves Lives, But Your Paperwork Saves You.

When we came out of the room, Dr. DAM instructed me" Welcome to the world of absurdity, Gupta. First of all, let us convey this to our head of unit, Dr. Modi, and ask him to remain absent throughout the inquiry as he has nothing to do with any of it. Second, go through the whole case paper and see if there is any gap. Make sure you don't alter anything in the case paper. Third, talk to all the staff in the Jain ward and also to Mrs. Nancy if they have any input about the husband of the sister and the union. Fourth, don't allow this inquiry to go over your head. Don't lose your cool, and don't speak a lot with anyone".

It was a long list, but an important one in the case of such inquiries. Do not alter anything on the case paper. This was perplexing. I thought if there was any gap, we could rectify it and make it watertight. But why he said no was confusing. So I asked this to Dr. Sharma, the third-year resident of Unit I. He was the most knowledgeable senior resident in the whole hospital. He explained" Gupta, when you alter, there are differences in pen, handwriting, and many other things. If someone catches you in this, then nothing can protect you from being pronounced guilty. **So in any case, never alter the case paper in such inquires. This was the most important golden rule I learned today**.

So then the day arrived when we were supposed to be present in front of the inquiry commission. When I and my professor entered the superintendent's room, there was a huge crowd. There were a municipal commissioner, a lawyer, other professors, a matron, the husband of the deceased, and a few others whom we could not recognize. So the commission began. The chairman of the inquiry was the Municipal Commissioner, who started" This is an inquiry to find out facts about the treatment given and about the reasons for the death of Mrs. Shah. She was also a senior staff member at this hospital. The inquiry will be headed by me, assisted by the superintendent, matron of the hospital, a lawyer, and a social worker."

Dr. DAM looked towards me as if he were telling me," What nonsense! The person who is responsible for the whole mess is going to assist. So now we are doomed, as we knew that this would be a one-sided inquiry". But I guess we have no way to escape. So I guess Sir decided to see what happens in due course.

Dr. DAM was called first. He went into a separate room, where he was asked about the sister's history and course of treatment. He has read the whole file, and since he was only taking rounds daily, he knew the whole progress. Now I understand why he said on day one not to allow Dr. Modi to take rounds on this patient. If, as per routine, they take rounds alternately, then Dr. DAM would have gaps in remembering the progress. In that case, Dr. Modi would also have been part of the inquiry.

After about half an hour, he came out. He looked tired but visibly angry. He saw me and said, "Dr. Gupta, you go in. Don't worry. Be relaxed and say what you are asked. Don't get nervous. You are just a witness, so don't worry". I felt a bit relieved to hear him. But I knew that my professor was in the dock for no fault of his. So I went in.

Commissioner "Yes, please sit. Tell us your name and designation."

"Sir, my name is Dr. Gupta, and I am a first-year resident in Unit 3 under Dr. Modi and Dr. DAM."

Commissioner" Oh, first year. Dr. Mukesh, why have you called him? He is just in his first year; how can he help us? Why harass him for this? We all know they are supposed to follow the treatment and advice in the first year. You should have called it "third-year resident of the unit".

Dr. Mukesh" Sorry,but he is the only resident that this unit has. And he was involved in management from day one under Mrs. Shah. So in fact, he knows all the things. ``

Commissioner with respect and sympathy"Ok, Doctor, tell me the whole progress of the sister from day one". I like a parrot depicted the whole story as it was from day 1 until her death.

Lawyer" So tell me, doctor, was the sister getting her injections at the right time? Since she suffered from such a contagious disease, were staff and you ready to give her proper care".

I felt a punch but still kept cool "Sir, from day one she got all the injections; all her reports were done on time. You can see in the case paper."

Lawyer "Yes, I can see that, but how can you be sure that what was written in the paper was actually given?

"Sir, if you see the case paper, there is a time written in front of every injection or medicine. So it is given at that time only."

Commissioner"No, no, you did not understand the question. He is asking, How are you sure that she got the injection or medicine at the right time or that she really got the medicine?"

"Sir, when medicine is given to any patient, the sister who gives it does a small sign on the time to depict that medicine given."

Lawyer"Still, there is a chance that she might not have gotten medicine."

I lost my control. "Sir, in that case, you can say this for every patient in this country. Even though we wrote, it is possible that staff did not give the medicine. Sorry, but that's not the way things work. You can ask the superintendent, sir. He is head of department also.``

Dr. Mukesh got angry' Dr., don't act smart. You don't need to ask any of us a question. We will ask questions".

Commissioner" I was going through the case papers. Why is it that the same medicines are written daily on the new page? Many days it appears you have just copied the previous day's page."

I felt like laughing, but with a smirk I replied, "Sir, once the treatment plan is fixed, the medicines remain the same daily. So we have to write a fresh prescription page daily for proper documentation and clarity."

Social worker" But then it is possible that your professor did not take sufficient rounds or missed the rounds, and so you copied the previous day's details."

I laughed this time"Sorry, maam, but every time our professor takes a round, the resident who gives him a round will write, seen by so and so professor. So please go through every day's case paper, and you will see that it is written on every page.

Social worker' But that could have been written by you despite your professor not coming."

I thought of giving an earful to all these people, but, "Sorry, maam, I don't have an answer to that."

The day ended with this inquiry. I really felt angry. But anger was taken over by the whole day's work that has suffered because of this inquiry. So I rushed back to my ward and worked like a donkey the whole day to finish the pending work. Again, the meal was not possible.

This inquiry went on for the next three months. Now the center of attention was only me. I would have been called almost 10 times after. Every time, I answered only absurd questions.

Commissioner" Who sent the report on HIV? Why was she transferred from the VIP room to the Jain ward? Why were various reports done outside in a private lab?

Lawyer" Who decided the therapy? Who decided on the reports? Why was treatment for HIV started after the western blot and not after the first report? Was this delay not responsible for the delay in treatment? Why was no other specialist called for the treatment?

Social worker" Was she given proper food in time? Does she know about her disease? How was the behavior of the staff and you with the patient?

I answered each one of these questions with a cool mind. As time passed, things became routine for me. So rather than being nervous, I was enjoying the learning process. I knew the treatment given, the decision taken in real time in case of an emergency, and all the actual thought during the day-to-day treatment had no value in this inquiry. The only thing that matters is the case paper. My professor, Dr. DAM, has always told me, "Gupta, **remember the golden rule. Always take rounds and write down the findings with a date and time. If you communicate with some relatives, try to mention their names in the case paper. In a court of law, your effort will not matter, but only the things written in the case paper will matter"**.

At one point, the investigation did cover the Superintendent's response and behavior. Commissioner asked" Dr. In our hospital, as far as I know, there is a rule of indenting medicines and reports for the needy and others. I see many of these reports and medicines were indented in Mrs. Shah's also. So tell me, did you get those medicines and reports on time? Did the superintendent do it promptly?"Luckily, my professor has told me not to tell the truth about indent and superintendent behavior. He said, "We will not say anything bad against the superintendent, as by proving him wrong we will only add to our problems."

So I said, "Sir, it was very prompt. We got all the medicines and reports on time."

It took almost three months to complete the inquiry. And the day of calling was always sudden, which led to a complete disturbance of the day-to-day schedule of mine, and above all, of my professor also

All Were Happy, But What About The Donkey?

My professor Dr. DAM was getting irritated day by day. So at the end of three months, when we were called again, he decided to do something about this. He said on that day, "Dr. Gupta, come on today; let's make this the last day of the inquiry. I guess we need to call the fox a fox". I felt frightened but excited about the events that were going to unfold. When we entered, the crowd was larger than the first day. All were present on day one. But apart from this, there were more senior staff and many media personnel. I came to know just before this meeting today that Dr. DAM was the brother of an influential local MLA in the city. So he has asked his brother to help him get media coverage during the inquiry. So there we were. Just as the commission was going to go into a separate room to start the proceedings, Dr. DAM got up from his seat. He said, "Respected committee members and others present, before you begin the proceedings, I want to say something. Please permit me."

The superintendent felt the punch, and as if he knew what was coming, he protested the move. But the husband of the deceased got up. He said, "I think it is ok if he is allowed to speak".

Commissioner, though a bit irritated, said, "Ok, Dr. DAM, but please be brief.'

Dr. DAM" Ladies and gentlemen, almost three months are over in this inquiry. And I wish to ask a few questions to 2 to 3 people in this room. Firstly, I want to ask the nursing matron and other senior staff present here. Do you have any complaints against our unit, which gave treatment to Mrs. Shah? You all were part of the day-to-day care of this patient. Do you think we have acted negligently?"

The commissioner almost shouted, "Dr., they are nobody to decide this. We are here to decide this".But by then Mrs. Nancy had risen and started her speech" Sir, let me say on behalf of all the staff here. We are very satisfied with the care you gave, especially to your resident. He was present almost 24 hours a day. "

Dr. DAM continued "Mr. Shah, I know you have lost your wife. I know you are angry about many things. But please tell me if you are angry with me and my unit. Do you think we were negligent in our treatment?

Mr Shah" Dr DAM and Dr Gupta frankly speaking, I'm thankful to you and your unit that I knew what my wife was suffering from. You have taken care of her like a sister. I have no complaints against you or your unit. That is what I have been telling this committee since day 1, but they are not listening."

There was a huge uproar in the crowd. They knew that something was wrong. Mr. Shah continued as if he had his voice back" It is the superintendent against whom I have a problem. He has been treating my wife for a year. He had done thousands of reports. He has given her so many medicines and injections. In fact, two to 3 times he has ordered the removal of fluid from the lungs as well. Whenever we asked him about the possible reasons, he would never give one. He would say it might be malaria, typhoid, tuberculosis, or whatnot. When we asked him why she was not recovering, he suggested that she was having psychological issues and had prescribed her medicine for that as well. I can show you all the papers. This admission under Dr. DAM, sir, has led to a diagnosis within one day. Then, after they have tried everything to treat it, the disease has already worsened until now.``

Commissioner "Don't worry, we will allow you to speak in due course. Then you can tell all these things."

Nursing matron" No sir, this is not done. I have been telling you all to call him and other staff for the last 2 months. We are just dragging the matter along. We have the answers from both doctors, and we have all the case papers. But instead of knowing the real issue, we are just dragging.``

So I guess the fire that my professor wanted to ignite has been ignited. The commissioner knew this, and one can see beads of perspiration on the superintendent's face. The lawyer and social worker were like bystanders who knew they could not do anything about this. Throughout the inquiry, they have tried to pin the blame on our unit.

The commissioner, looking at the gravity of the situation, adjourned the meeting. We all left, but Dr. DAM prepared a second assault. He has asked his brother to make matters political. So for the next few days, both the media and political members of his brother's party kept the kettle boiling. They raised the questions that finally made the commissioner dismiss the inquiry against our unit, and he made Mr. Shah and Superintendent sit together. They came up with a compromise formula. Mr. Shah was taken back to work after the inquiry was dismissed. Dr. Mukesh said in writing that he will bear all the expenses of the education of both kids until college. And that he will release Mrs. Shah's pension and other perks immediately.

A long ordeal was finally over. Dr. DAM was happy that he could pull this off smoothly. Mr.Shah was happy that he got his job and money for the education of his kids. Staff unions were happy that they could pressurize the corporation and hospital to penalize the culprit. As far as I am concerned, I felt happy for these people, but this event became a watershed for me. The superintendent made it his aim in life to make my residency difficult. As everyone knows, I was all alone in the unit, so my professor got me help from the superintendent on every emergency day to get an extra hand to help. But after this event, that hand vanished. He made sure that I remained alone. The indents in our unit dried up as he delayed signing them until late. Those staff members who were close to him unleashed their own terror in the unit. When we finish our first year, the second year is for rotation. This year we are assigned duties with super-specialized units like cardiology, neurology, gastroenterology, nephrology, and endocrinology. This was most important for any medical doctor. During this time, we learned so much about different organs and their diseases. But the assignment came through the superintendent's office. So he made sure that I did not get an important rotation from the above. In fact, I was given 6 months of endocrinology and then 3 months of cardiology and neurology, respectively. Out of these 3 months of cardiology, I was given to a different peripheral center, which actually forced me to leave my hostel for that period. So I guess the incident led to huge educational problems for me.

When I look back today, I feel that it was a blessing in disguise for me. Learning these things in medical practice, like communication, writing case papers,doing what is right for the patient, and relatives' own selfish agendas, makes a lot of difference. Since I was all alone, I did all the work, like morning rounds, collecting blood reports, giving rounds to my professors, post-round follow-up things, attending OPD, and attending all emergencies. Along with that, one more thing happened. The majority of the staff started respecting me and helping me in my day-to-day work.

The respect and pampering that were available to 3rd-year residents were available to me from the first year itself. So I guess, apart from the superintendent, others helped me in my residency.

My first year was definitely hard work. During this time, apart from these few events, Ahmedabad also had to face two major disasters. One was the flood of a lifetime. It rained for four continuous days, which led to major flooding. Because of this, a huge number of casualties came, and later on, disease endemics also started. The wards were full, so patients were given a down cot, which means floor, to sleep on and take medicines. It lasted almost a month, and during this period, I and my colleagues learned a lot of medicine. There were patients of all ages with all different diseases and complications. So the burden of disaster was proving to be a learning curve for us, which the majority of physicians learn in 8 to 10 years. Later, Ahmedabad faced the worst malaria endemic, which for the first time in the history of malaria showed to be resistant malaria. Almost every professor said that they had never seen such complicated malaria or deaths due to malaria. The medicines did not work, reports were not helping, and a huge number of patients required lots of blood and product transfusions, dialysis, and what not. But every unit in the hospital and even in the city lost more than 30% of the patients. This was stressful. We have learned to deal with the physical and mental stress of work burden and complications in patients, but for the first time, we were learning to continue working even with so much death and suffering around. Every day we tried to find a new solution to treat, and if anyone said their technique worked, we all started following that. But nature has made it a point to prove that it can be deadly if we don't follow the basic laws of hygiene. So the first year was like 10 years for us colleagues. But still, when it ended, almost everyone was disturbed. We knew we would be separated for one year now. Few will be in the same hospital, and few will be sent to different hospitals in town. But for at least a year, our day-to-day meetings, eating together, reading together, and going out together will stop. We have established a strong bond between the eight of us. We were told stories of depression when we joined residency. We were told it would be very hard and would take away sleep and food. We were told that many ran away and also suffered from disease during the residency. But somehow, after joining, we became resistant to stress. We decided on a plan. We made sure that none of us would work without a proper breakfast. If anyone was free and was in the hospital, then we would assist one another. If there is a good case to study, we will present it in front of each other and try to learn from each other's experience. We made sure that we had at least one meal together with as many of us present as possible. We went out for walks around the hospital frequently, and we went to movies together frequently. We had made a group of colleagues of different specialties to make life easier around us. Every professor and every senior resident knew us personally within a few months, and it was the first time in the history of the hospital that the professor took rounds with the help of residents of any unit present. So in short, we tried to ease out our stress with as many people around us as possible. And so when the first year ended, almost everyone praised us for our progress and predicted that when we returned in the third year as senior residents, it would be the golden period of the medical ward. So with a sense of achievement, pride, and a bit of sadness, we went on for your second year.

You Are My Competitors, So Remain An Average Doctor. Absurd And Shameful

So then began my second year of residency. A year of rotation. I was punished for my involvement in the Mrs. Shah medical issue and the inquiry that followed. Dr. Shah, the superintendent, has assigned me only 3 rotations in place of 5. My first rotation was in neurology, then I spent 3 months at Shardaben General Hospital, which was 5 km away from this hospital, and so I was forced to leave the hostel for that period. And later, he gave me six months of continuous endocrinology rotation. To date, none of the residents in the recent past has done more than 2 months of endocrinology.

So neurology it was. This ward was on the fourth floor of the hospital. In fact, the fourth floor was dedicated to neurology and nephrology. Mrs. Nancy"Guptaji, you are going to the fourth floor in the ward of neurology. There are two senior staff members there, Mrs. Shabnam and Mrs. Patil. Both of them are very close to professors in neurology and nephrology. Don't fight with them; otherwise, you will not learn anything from the professors."

Mrs. Dharti" Sister, what are you telling? This fellow will never do that. You know him; he will definitely enter into a fight if he feels like it. And if a patient is going to suffer, then fighting is inevitable".

Everyone around the table laughed. Mrs. Nancy" Don't worry, we are just one floor down. And you will be coming to this ward anyhow, daily. So we will sort out any issues. So go and learn."

Mrs. Nancy continued" Now you will see how super specialists work, behave, act, and conduct themselves. You will see three big shots in the unit. Dr. Acharya is the head of the department. He has an air of arrogance, but he is the most humble. He is a no-nonsense guy. He will come and take rounds daily at the same time. He will teach if you ask. Even in OPD, he will see one patient at a time."

Mrs. Tambe" Do you remember what he did to one of the political people in his OPD? He was seeing a patient when this fellow barged in with arrogance. And he then started talking to Dr. Acharya out of turn. Dr. Acharya got up and politely asked him to go out of the OPD. But that fellow kept talking absurdly. Then Dr. Acharya lost his cool, caught him by the collar, and took him out of OPD. He then categorically gave an order to the receptionist to not allow this fellow inside his cabin". That fellow created a huge rukus then and there. He went to the superintendent and even to the commissioner of the town. But still, Dr. Acharya said only one thing "I am not his slave. If he doesn't respect me, then in my cabin I am the king. Next time he does this, I will file a case against him."

Mrs. Nancy, "Dr. Acharya always says one thing, Sister if I don't have self-respect, then no one will give me respect. And there is nothing wrong with fighting for self-respect."

Mrs. Tambe" Nancy, see the light in this fellow's eyes. Let's bet that Gupta will have a fight in the first week itself. Now he knows that his head of department is Dr. Acharya and that he agrees to fight for the right thing."

Everyone, including me, laughed. But I said, "Sister, frankly, it's not like I like fighting, but maybe I have an issue with my temper. I will try to control."

On that also, as if I had said the joke of the century, almost everyone on the table and around laughed.

I asked, "But sister, you have described only one professor in neurology. What about others?"

Mrs. Nancy" The associate professor is Dr. Jain. Try to stay away from him. Rather than teaching you anything, he might take away all that you have studied. He believes that by teaching students, they are preparing for future competition. So why teach them and make them experts? Let them be simple MBBS so that they can refer everything to them.``

Mrs. Tambe" And moreover, he is very much against Dr. Joshi. He is your assistant professor in neurology. He is young, dynamic, and very student-friendly. If you remain with him for a year, he can easily make you a good clinician."

"But why is Dr. Jain against Dr. Joshi?"

Nancy sister "Dr. Jain sees Dr. Joshi as his competitor, and since Dr. Joshi is really good, he feels that he will take away all his patients. He did all to prevent Dr. Joshi from joining our hospital."

Neurology itself is a demanding subject. Half of the patients, despite being diagnosed, cannot recover due to a lack of medicines or the possibility of surgeries. So patients always thought that it was a useless branch that only sucked money and gave no results. The history and examination of the patient themselves can take an hour. So just think about what will happen on emergency days. Over that, every alternate day I will have an emergency as we have two residents in rotation, and on that, this internal politics of professors

I shouted, "You people are here to help or make me nervous."

Now everyone laughed as if they enjoyed my nervousness.

So on day one, when I went to Ward 14 on the fourth floor, I saw Dr. Patel standing at the desk. He was a fellow resident in rotation. He has come from Shardaben Government Hospital, a sister hospital of the corporation. There were also postgraduate courses going on at another hospital, i.e., the LG government hospital. I knew him because of his stories of a bad temper and I don't care attitude that were famous in all three hospitals. He has entered into big fights with seniors and even a few professors for petty reasons. So I felt a moment of despair seeing him. He was the last thing I wanted with me in neurology rotation, along with all the stories that my sisters have told me about the department. But again, do I have any choice? So I went ahead and introduced myself. Surprisingly, he knew me. He said, "Doctor, I know you because of the HIV case and its fallout."

I" Oh ok". I was a bit overwhelmed by his behavior and attitude, and so I somehow felt worried. We were told about all the patients present in the neurology department by the sister. We were handed a list of all the references that the neurology department had from the hospital. It was a huge task on its own. Dr. Patel gave a few cuss words to the sister and looked at me as if he were saying, "Who cares? Let the professors come; we will go with them in rounds, and then after, we will see what is to be done".

I asked him, "Dr. Patel, now that we have a list, let's divide the work. If you wish, you can take rounds of the neurology ward, and I will go to see references of the patients, or else the other way around is also ok with me."

Patel" Guptaji, chill. Let's skip this part today. We will tell them that we got the list just now. We will move with professors and take a round with them only."

The way I have done my first year of residency, this was unheard of, or, let's say, unacceptable to me. I will always like to be prepared for rounds. I have understood that knowing the patients before my professor comes gives me more opportunities to learn from every patient. But here is a person who wanted to take rounds with professors as if he were a newly appointed professor. I said, "No boss. This is not how I do residency. You choose what you want. Then, if you wish, take the round or else sit and wait for the professors. I will definitely go and see patients on my part". So I guess on the first day I already developed a sort of friction with the colleague. This also means that for the next three months I will have no help from him if there is any work stress, any complications, or any social issues. But then, last year taught me a lot.

I went on to see the patients who were referred to the neurology department. They were all over the hospital. So for the first time, I was going to all different departments alone as a senior resident. I went to the surgical ward, neurosurgical ward, gynecology ward, gastro ward, cardiothoracic ward, and cardiology ward. Then, after this, when I entered the medical wards of my parent unit, there was an air of pride and a bit of arrogance that creeped in. I went to the desk and said with authority, "Sister, tell me the bed number of patients who are referred for neurology reference. And also send one junior staff member with a case paper."

The moment my sentence finished, senior staff saw me as if I had said some abuse "Guptaji, still, you are what you were in your first year. It's just the first day of rotation, and you are acting as if you are the boss. Even your boss doesn't come and demand these things. You have a list of patients with names, units, and bed numbers. Go find yourself; if there is no case paper, then come and get it from here. And still, junior staff are not available, as they were not when you were here as a junior in your first year."

Another shouted, "Keep your foot on the ground."

I really came back thrashing on the floor. I went ahead and did what I was told. It consumed a lot of my time. I did not want to get late for rounds with the professors on day one itself. So I left without seeing all the referred patients and rushed towards the fourth floor. Luckily, the professor came around 5 minutes after I arrived. Though I was not prepared for the rounds, I felt I was more prepared than my fellow colleague, who was actually gossiping with junior staff when I came back.

It was one of the most exhaustive rounds to date. It lasted for three hours. There were three professors, and each had their work divided systematically. Dr. Acharya took rounds in medical wards where he saw the references. Since I have seen only a few patients, I could not answer a lot of questions. Since this was the first day, he seemed lenient. But I felt let down by myself. But his walk itself was a terror. He had a 6.2-foot, 100-kg body and walked like an army major. When he talked, it was very polite and courteous.

Then another was about Dr. Jain. He took rounds in Ward 14 on the fourth floor. This was actually a neurology ward, and the patients were admitted under our care only. But since our great Dr. Patel has not taken any patients there, Dr. Jain immediately knew that we did not know anything about the patients there. For almost the next 40 minutes or so, Dr. Patel and I got to hear sarcastic statements. He kept abusing us sarcastically in front of relatives, ward boys, nurses, and even bystanders.

"You people are of no use. A day before, you should have come and taken over this patient."

"I am sure you would have come here only in the morning. You people just stroll here like in a park and then after 3 years of residency and getting a degree, you will come and practice and take away our patients."

"Many of you will be rich, and so will start big nursing homes and take away our hard-earned practice."

The tirade of words went on until the end of the round. I could now realize the intensity of the words told to me by the ward 10 sister just the other day. So in the next three months, we will be facing this. We don't know how much we may learn from him, but we are sure of what we will hear from him. His tirade actually did one good thing. Dr. Patel" Dr. Gupta, this is serious ragging. I think we need to work together and prevent as much ragging as possible. We need to cover for each other". So I guess calamity united us.

Then came the fresh breeze of air. Now came the round with Dr. Joshi. When he walked into the ward, he had a different aura. He looked so kind, with a smile on his face and a beard. He had dressed so well, with a white shirt and a tie. When he reached us, he welcomed us. Dr. Patel" That's first; a professor welcoming us is so good."

Instantly, we became fans. During the whole round he taught us, his basics were so clear, and he knew what teaching we needed on the first day. He took almost 1 and a half hours to see six patients, but each and every one was thoroughly examined and seen. After the round, we both talked only about him.

Dr. Patel" I have not seen anyone taking such a round. He is so thorough".

I" Yes. His questions, follow-up questions, examination and interpretation of each thing, and finally the possible diagnosis are so strong."

I continued" In fact, after the whole process, he could diagnose the disease without any investigation. It appeared he wanted those investigations to confirm his diagnosis".

Dr. Patel "Dr. Jain took hardly 3 to 4 minutes to finish seeing a patient. For every patient, he advised a long list of investigations. At the end of the investigation, at least something will come, and then he will boost his chances of diagnosing rare diseases. ``

But by seeing his list of investigations, I guess we cannot treat any middle-class patient. Only the reports would cost in the range of 20 to 30 thousand rupees."

Then we remembered what Dr. Joshi told us at the end of the round; in fact, he told us many things.

First, there are fast neurologists and slow neurologists. The fast neurologists are costly, and they get fame as they diagnose disease in a day or two. The slow neurologist takes a step-by-step approach and so may look confused."

Secondly, when you prescribe medicine, you should know the side effects of every medicine. The effects are known to all, but if you don't know the most common side effects, then you will hurt your patient more".

"**Third, if your history and examination are not matching, then it means either of them is wrong. In that case, revisit every detail to fill the gap.**

Dr. Patel and I, after the round, would have repeated these three statements almost 50 times in front of everyone who met us that day. We were so impressed by him that we dreamed of remaining with him for the rest of his two years of residency. But I guess that's a dream.

So the first day gave us a glimpse of what was to come for the next three months. But teaching was huge, and so we both enjoyed the rotation. It was first on the list, but it shaped the whole clinical practice.

"Bro, the clinical exam that we are learning here is going to help us pass the exams. Every long case in the exam has neurology things."

Dr. Patel" You are right. But frankly, what we are learning is going to help us practice smoothly and confidently. A large number of patients in practice will have headaches, strokes, leg pain, parkinsonism, memory loss, and so on."

I learned one more thing from Dr. Joshi yesterday. I am now referring to all his rules as golden rules. He said that **in practice, if you are going to work as a physician, you should know which patients need to be referred to a superspecialist. You can't refer every patient with a headache to a neurologist.** He is so right."

Patel" Yes. This is true for all things."

So such discussions became common between both of us. We discussed difficult cases and practiced various clinical exams. Dr. Joshi was so much into teaching that he started taking lectures every 15 days. So I guess we were on the right track. We were both becoming independent in taking decisions, and if proven right, at least Dr. Acharya and Dr. Joshi were always there to praise. If proven wrong, then Dr. Joshi would guide. Dr. Jain remained same and his sarcasm and showing us inferiority continued.

I Am Also Human But Still A Doctor. Empathy And Care Are A Must.

It was Tuesday, and it was my emergency. In the OPD, I was sitting with Dr. Joshi. A young girl came in with her parents. Father" Sir, my daughter Shyamli has been suffering from fever for a month. She has also lost weight and is not eating properly.``

As usual, Dr. Joshi was thorough. He asked pertinent questions" Does she have headache, vomiting, giddiness, loss of consciousness, weakness in any arm or leg, abdominal pain, cough, breathlessness, and so on?"

Father" She has had a fever, weight loss, headache, and nausea for 1 month. She did not have a cough or breathlessness. Since the last 5 days, her headache has increased."

Mother"Sir, she has been vomiting for 3 days and has not eaten anything since then. Yesterday she fell down while going to the toilet."

Dr. Joshi asked me, "Dr. Gupta, what should be your next question to them?"

I was taken aback a little, but I knew his style and was not nervous, so I asked her father, "Who saw her falling down or who attended her then?"

Her mother said she did. So I asked her, "Did her eyes roll up? Does she have jerky movements in her legs and arms? Was there any froth in the mouth? Did she urinate?"

Her mother replied positively to all the questions. So I turned to sir and said, "Sir, it looks like a seizure."

Dr. Joshi"Yes, primarily, it looks like this. But you should also ask about the time of recovery How was her memory? Was there any headache after waking up?"

When asked, Mother replied, "Sir, she did not remember anything about the event; she was crying because of a headache after becoming conscious."

Dr. Joshi and I examined her meticulously. Sir asked me to note all my findings. He then advised the parents to admit their child to the ward for further investigation and treatment. The father said, "Sir, give me some medicine. We have come from faraway places and have not arranged for admission. We will come after 5 to 7 days."

I have never seen Sir get irritated until now. But he said a bit loudly, "Brother, your daughter is critical, and she does not have that much time. She has an infection in her brain, and if we don't find the type of infection and start treatment at the earliest, she may go into a coma or die".

Still, the father persisted "Sir, please give me some medicine. I have another kid at home, and then we have a function next week. So we will come after a few days."

This time the mother shouted at her husband, "What are you talking about? Don't you listen; the doctor is telling you she may go into a coma or die. You are thinking of functions. If she lives, we will do many such things. Already, you and your work have delayed the treatment. I am telling you that she is suffering, and we should come to Ahmedabad at the earliest. But you and your work."

She continued" If you want, you can go; I will stay with my daughter. Sir, you admit her".

So finally, a social fight ended well for the kid, and she was admitted. Sir has advised her to get a lumbar puncture first and then give her an antibiotic and steroid injection. So I asked, "Sir, but lumbar puncture will happen after an hour or so. Why don't we start the injections? She can have relief immediately, then."

Dr. Joshi "She might have temporary relief, but we may lose the important diagnosis. Always remember that the diagnosis should not be compromised if possible. If you give antibiotics and steroids, then the cerebrospinal fluid exam may come back wrong or negative. So do LP first and then injections."

I understood the therapy, and I asked the ward boy to take the patient to ward 14 immediately. I called the sister there to keep the LP tray ready and also get the tubes to collect the CSF fluid. Sir asked me to accompany the patient so that there would be no delay. He continued his OPD alone. None of the other professors would have done that. They would have finished the OPD with residents sitting across from them. This would have delayed the process.

I accompanied the patient to Ward 14. After the patient settled, I was ready for the LP. I have already done multiple procedures and was confident in the procedure. The sister came to the parents to get their consent. She asked her father to sign a paper that "doctor is going to perform the LP. The procedure is well explained to me in my language. He has told us all the risks. So I agree and allow the doctor to do the procedure".

I explained everything to them, and they agreed while we were on the way from OPD. But now they did a sudden turn around. This time the mother said, "Doctor, we don't want you to do LP on my daughter. This procedure can lead to leg paralysis and cause pain for my kid. So we will not allow it. You inject and do all the other reports."

I tried to reason with them" Madam, if we don't do this and don't send a CSF report, then we will never know if there is a bacterial infection, a viral infection, or tuberculosis. Doing this will help us know which medicines to give and for what duration."

This time, Father shouted, "Doctor, you people are trapping us. You say one thing and then say something else. Your sir told us to admit to giving injections. Now you want to hurt my kid."

It was almost 1.30 p.m. This patient has already consumed two and a half hours of mine from OPD until now. So hunger, the illiteracy of parents, their false accusation of trapping them, and the kids' critical condition led to a burst of anger in me. I lost my temper and shouted, "How dare you say this to me? My unit and I have been trying to help you for the last 2 hours. I have not eaten anything till now and am doing the procedure at the earliest possible time so that we can give her injections. At first, you were not ready to admit her, and now you want me to do unethical things with your kid. When you don't care for your kid, then why should I waste my time on her? Let her suffer.``

Saying this, I rushed out of the room and went to my PG hostel. I went directly to the canteen to eat my lunch. But while eating, I suddenly felt a punch. I felt very low. I could not eat my lunch further. For the first time, I felt ashamed of myself. I felt sorry for the kid and even for the parents. I realized how health illiterate we are as a country. Even the most educated don't understand health issues. This was a simple family where the collective education in the family was up to the 8th standard. I thought, it's my duty to remain calm. They may not agree, but I need to be persistent. I am the one who knows what can happen to the patient. I need to tell them and make them understand the gravity.``

I left my lunch and rushed back to Ward 14. When the staff saw me, she said, "Why are you here now? You just tell us what injections are to be given, and we will start. If they are not ready for the procedure, then why waste time? Leave them to their fate."

I said, "No, sister. I will not do that. Let me give it one more try."

I went into the room. Seeing me, the father rushed to me with folded hands. "Sorry, doctor Sahab. I am a village person. I don't understand that you are doing all this for my child."

I calmly asked them to sit. I explained the whole procedure, the importance of the result, and how it will help doctors decide the treatment. They both agreed and said, "Sir, frankly, after you left, Shyamli told us, Don't worry, Mummy, Papa, I will do it. Let the doctor do it; he is doing it for me only."

Mother" Seeing the courage of Shyamli, we also agreed to the procedure. So please, sir, do it, and please see to it that there is no harm to her.

Her final sentence gave me a jitter. All the confidence vanished, and the sense of the final exam came in. I prayed that all would go well. I passed the procedure with flying colors. After that, reports were sent, and injections were given immediately. Both my parents and Shyamli thanked me with folded hands. With a sense of achievement, I went back to the hostel. But the lunch hour was gone, but still, the stomach was full with thanks from all three of them. So I just closed my eyes and slept in my room. The lesson was well learned. **We are doctors, and it is we who know the disease and its sequelae. Also, not all patients or relatives are the same. But we need to be cool, calm, and graceful to help patients and their relatives reach the best possible decisions. These decisions will help them recover, and retrospectively, they will always thank us.**

By evening, I got the report of the CSF, and as suspected by Dr. Joshi, it turned out to be tuberculosis meningitis. I talked to the parents"Sir, your daughter is having Tb, and it has affected the brain and its layers. Because of this, there is swelling inside, which leads to headaches, vomiting, seizures, and loss of consciousness. They got worried, and so they asked,

"Sir, we don't know all this stuff." Just tell us she will live. Please do all you can to save her."

Though unsure of the future, I said, "Sir, don't worry. We have all the medicines for this disease. She will recover. But she will have to be in the hospital for a longer time, and she will have to take medicines for more than a year."

Mother "Sir, you just saved her; I will do whatever you tell me and for whatever duration you tell me."

I know I have not informed them of all the risks that she has, both immediately and at a later date. But I took that liberty, as they have already suffered mentally a lot today. So I informed Dr. Joshi about the report, and he started medicine for her. He asked me to study the disease, investigations, their interpretations, medicines to save lives, and medicines to treat the disease. I knew it was a lengthy subject, but because of his clinical approach, I have learned a lot of practical details about the disease. So today was a very fruitful day. I went for my first complete meal of the day after finishing the rest of the work. I discussed the whole event with my colleagues, and they also learned what I did through my description.

Dr. Patel" Our rotation in neurology has really become a fruitful exercise. We are learning so much."

I" Yes, we had similar patients in our medical ward also in the first year. But the way of looking at them, the questions we asked then, the reports and their interpretations, and even the treatment are so different. In fact, because of the overload, we took a shortcut. We referred them to the neurology department. Then we just did what they advised without thinking why they did so".

Dr. Patel" I guess that's the reason this rotation system was developed in our curriculum. This is giving us exposure to different specialties so that when we go out and practice, we know the basics."

"Yes, as our sir, Dr. Joshi, says, as physicians, we should know all the diseases and their basics. Along with that, it is our job to see to whom to refer."

Own The Responsibility. Respect The Colleague. Otherwise, There Is No Respect.

It was Friday, and the emergency was with Dr. Patel, and the professor in charge that day was Dr. Jain. Normally, on emergency days, we both take rounds in the morning and finish our respective jobs after rounds. Then, after rounds, the person on emergency roll call remains on call for any call. The other person is free. So either we study, we go out, or we go home for that day. The person on emergency call will see every patient for whom there is a reference or who gets admitted. If he wants to get advice from the professor, then the professor on call will help him on the phone. If there is a critical case, then the professor comes and personally sees the patient at any time of the day and provides expert advice.

Around midnight, Dr. Patel got a call from the gynecology department. It was about a patient who was admitted to the ward and who had delivered a child that morning. After delivery, the patient had seizures and also went into a semi-conscious state. So the doctor in the gynecology department has given an emergency referral to neurology. Dr. Patel promptly responded to the call. After assessing the patient, he thought of consulting the professor as it was a critical case. So he went on to the call center of the hospital and called Dr. Jain. He tried for almost 15 minutes, but Dr. Jain did not pick up the call even after so many calls. So finally, Patel called the next in line, Dr. Joshi. Sir promptly picked up the call as usual.

Dr. Patel 'Sir, I have come to see an emergency reference in the Gynecology department. It is a young female who has gone into a postpartum seizure. What should I do?"

Dr. Joshi" But Patel, today is Dr. Jain's emergency; why are you calling me?"

Dr. Patel"Sir, I tried Dr. Jain, sir, for almost 15 minutes, but he is not picking up the call. So since time is of the essence, I called you."

Dr Joshi" Oh. Then it is ok."

He asked many questions regarding her history, examination, type of delivery, type of anesthesia or medicine given in the last 24 hours, her antenatal period, blood pressure, and sugar. He also inquired about her past deliveries and so on. After that, Dr. Joshi meticulously advised certain reports and medicine on an immediate basis. And he also told him, "Dr. Patel, don't leave the patient's ward till she settles. See for yourself that injections are given at the proper dose. Also, see that you collect the reports. Once she settles, transfer this patient to our side in the emergency ward."

Though it was midnight and Dr. Patel was tired and sleepy, he felt a surge of adrenaline. He knew that the night was long today, but if he does what is being told and if the patient recovers and wakes up, then it will be job satisfaction. So like a disciplined soldier, he went to the gynecology ward and did what was told. By morning, the patient's seizures had stopped, she started responding to verbal commands, and she was transferred to the emergency ward under the neurology unit.

In the morning, we both completed the rounds as per normal, and then we reached the clock tower. This was a landmark of this hospital, from where all entered the hospital. So daily we have to reach here, and as and when professors arrive, one or both of us accompany them. It was also a rule that if any patient was critical, rounds would start in the emergency room. So unfortunately, the first person to arrive that day was Dr. Jain. So as per protocol, we took him to the emergency room.

When we reached the emergency room, Dr. Patel started telling us about the history.

Dr. Patel "Sir, this is a 30-year-old female, Tina Shah, who was admitted to the gynecology ward for delivery. She delivered her baby on Friday morning through normal delivery."

Dr. Jain interrupted in between" So why is the patient in the emergency room? Why are we taking this route? Is this a reference to us? If this is a reference, why are we in the emergency room first? We need to see our patient first. And you know, I have a known patient who is admitted under us in ward 14."

Dr. Patel" That's what I am telling you, sir. She had a seizure, and she went into a semi-conscious state. We were referred on an emergency basis yesterday at midnight. I went in, saw her, and transferred her to the emergency room."

Dr. Jain shouted badly" But who are you to transfer her? How dare you take matters into your own hands?

Dr. Patel, though angry, gave a calm reply "Sir, I called you for almost 15 minutes, but you did not pick up the call."

Dr. Jain" Now to hide your mistake, you are blaming me. You never called me. I did not receive any calls."

Dr. Patel's anger was building, but he still replied, "Sir, what benefit will that give me? I did call you. Then, when you did not pick up, I called the next in line, Dr. Joshi.

Dr. Jain" You are a lazy fellow. You knew if you had to ring, then I would have ordered you some investigations and medicines, and you would have lost your sleep. So instead, you took the easy way out and shifted the patient to the ER."

Now Dr. Patel was ready to burst. He has called Dr. Joshi and, frankly, has not left the patient's bed till morning. And still he was blamed for negligence and laziness.

I saw his back; he had already made a fist as if to hit the professor. I thought that would be the end of our career and I would get punished for just being a bystander." So I immediately caught his hand from behind. He tried to free himself, but I kept my pressure. Dr. Patel continued" Sir, I am sorry to say, but you are wrong. I did call you, but you didn't pick up the call at night. So I have no option but to call Dr. Joshi. He did advise me on various things, and frankly, I went to my hostel to freshen up only in the morning once the patient settled. I was up the whole night. You can ask relatives."

Dr. Patel "Sir, if you want, you can ask Dr. Joshi. He will prove my point."

Dr. Jain" It is Dr. Joshi who has made you people worse. He has pampered you people, but he does not know what you will do to his and our practice after coming in private."

Now I also felt an urge, but I kept my cool as my career was in line. Just when Dr. Patel was looking like he would burst into anger and assault or abuse Dr. Jain, we saw Dr. Joshi enter the emergency room. I really felt relieved to see him. Dr. Jain was taken aback by his entry. Dr. Patel" Good morning, sir. This is the same patient that I called you.

Dr. Joshi "Oh, Ok. I guess she looks well and awake. It's good that you worked hard to help her recover. So what are her vitals and reports in the morning?"

Dr. Jain "Dr. Joshi, did this fellow call you at night? He is lying that he called me."

Dr. Joshi" He did call me. And whether he called you or not is difficult for me to say. But he did work very hard to save the patient's life.

Dr. Jain" But he is lying and insulting me. He embarrassed me in front of all the staff and patients' relatives."

Dr. Patel" But I only told you facts, sir. I did not insult you. And I did call you."

Dr. Jain "See, he is still lying. A liar cannot be in my unit. I will complain that these two people should be immediately removed from the neurology department."

Dr. Joshi"Sir, calm down. They are just residents. Please have a large heart and forgive them.

Dr. JainThese are regular offenders. They have an air of arrogance. They behave as if we are residents and they are professors. I cannot tolerate all this. I will definitely talk to the superintendent, Dr. Mukesh".

The matter settled, and we moved for further rounds. But this instance suggested that your colleague can prove you wrong and that your hard work can be trivialized by a stroke of ego. So maybe this incident made us realize the value of a good colleague or a good professor. Whether you help or don't is another matter, but your ego should not be bigger than a mountain. Lessons learnt. But one thing was sure with all such incidents, respect for Dr. Jain was fast reaching the baseline.

Nothing Is Better Than Nature, The Finest Teacher And The Finest University On Earth.

It was the 26th of January 2001. It was my emergency, and it was also a holiday. So that means there was no OPD and no rounds. So on such days, we were supposed to take rounds and inform the designated professor of the condition of the patients. The fellow who had been off would not even come for morning rounds. If there were private patients, i.e., the professor's personal patient, then the condition was informed to that professor only. So though I was on holiday, my work was tremendous as I was supposed to take rounds of all the patients, see all the referred patients, see the emergency patients, and also inform every professor of the designated patients. So for any resident, holidays were more hard work as professors and fellow residents were all on vacation. So Dr. Patel, I guess, would be sleeping in his house after a long night's party. And here I was in the hospital at 830 in the morning.

I went to the emergency room first and took the rounds, and after writing down the notes, I went to the fourth floor ward no. 14. I was taking my routine rounds. While taking the blood pressure of an elderly female patient, I suddenly felt as if I had giddiness. It seemed as if everything was rotating. But then the aged female shouted loudly that everything was moving and shaking. I shouted back," It's nothing. You have giddiness". But then everything really started shaking violently. The building was also shaking. There were loud shouts everywhere, and people started running in panic and fear. I also felt the fear of dying for the first time in my life. I ran towards the bridge that was there on the fourth floor that connected this building to the adjacent building. But the moment I stepped on the bridge, I saw a big crack occur in the middle. I knew it would fall, and so I shouted for everyone to go back to the building. Luckily, no one was injured then. Now I have only one way to get out of the building, and that is through the stairs. So we all ran towards the stairs and started going down the floors rapidly. There was loud panic shouting everywhere. Many shouted, saying that it was a possible attack by Pakistan. In both countries,

I guess if any big disaster happens, it is customary to blame the other. But I wondered how they could shake the buildings during an attack. Even if they attacked, they would do that by bombing. The only thing that can shake buildings or the earth is an atom bomb. The thought itself gave me a shiver. But then finally, someone shouted that it was an earthquake. And this made all things clear. When I reached the second floor I saw a few of my fellow colleagues. We got together and started going down. Suddenly I shouted, "Hey, what will happen to our immobile patients and those on ventilators? Almost everyone except one stood still in between. Many of the patients pushed us aside, and one of us almost fell down. We stepped aside in the corner and saw each other. We knew what we were supposed to do. So we rushed towards the wards to see if there were any bedridden patients. We tried to gather as many ward boys who had the courage to help and started evacuating the immobile patients with the help of their relatives and other bystanders. The moment of panic was now taken over by a sense of duty. Many non-paramedics stood to help. So slowly, every ward and ICU were screened, and bedridden patients were evacuated. The most difficult part was for those on ventilators. Their machines have stopped working due to a power failure.

When we reached the ICU, the scene over there was shocking. The patients on ventilators were gasping for air. There were tubes in their mouths, and the machine was not working. So neither the brain helped them breathe nor did the machine give them breath. It was like God and machines were choking them to death.

Relative of ICU bed 1" Hey doctor, please help my husband. He will die. He is not breathing. Please help."

Doctor 1 rushed to the bed. He saw all of us as if asking what to do. He was a surgical resident who had just joined his first year and had absolutely no knowledge about ventilators. So I shouted, "Doctor, just remove the machine connection from the tube."

He shouted back, "But then the patient will die if I cut him from the machine". I shouted back, "Doctor, but the machine is killing him as it has no power supply to provide breathing. So just do what I say."

In fact, like relative 1, almost all the relatives on all 10 beds were shouting, praying, and pleading with us to save their near and dear ones. The scene was like something from a horror movie or a Nazi Germany movie, where people were shouting and pleading for help when they knew they would die. So I shouted loudly for all the medical personnel standing there "All of you listen. Take an ambu bag from the cabinet. Take an oxygen tube. Attach the oxygen tube to the oxygen cylinder near the beds. Now attach one end to the ambu bag. Now remove the machine connection from the patient's tube. After that, join the ambu bag to the tube. Now push the ambu bag gradually and systematically."

So everyone followed these steps and did what I told them. Once we all saw the proper expansion of the chest of every patient, I shouted back, this time to relatives standing near the bed' All of you whose relatives are on the ventilator, please listen carefully."

The shaking got over after 15 minutes of it starting. Though there was an environment of fear, panic, and confusion everywhere, at least the fear in us doctors and paramedics was a bit low. So I said, "Look at the person pushing the bag and providing the breath to your relative. Now you have to do this until we shift them to a safe place or electricity comes. Don't worry; it is very easy. But we are low in numbers, and we need to be in many places to save people. So now learn and do it yourself."

So I could see things that were never imagined, where the life of the person was kept in the hands of relatives who knew nothing about medical equipment. But so were the times, which were making us learn things not in the books. Disaster management was not in any curriculum, but I guess today we learned how nature could be the best professor and the best book. It was giving all of us first-hand training.

So once this issue settled, a few of us remained there to observe and manage any eventuality. This was necessary as not all were there for ventilator treatment, but many had other requirements that, if not met on time, could lead to death or deterioration of health.

The rest of us went to the ground floor. The moment we reached the clock tower, we saw chaos and rickshaws, cars, and ambulances all around. A huge number of people were coming in with injuries and shock, and maybe a few were even dead. And frankly, since it was a national holiday, manpower in the hospital was also limited. The superintendent was not there, and when one of us called him, he said he was busy helping his family settle down, so he would take time to come there. The nursing staff and ward boys on duty were panicking, thinking about their families at home. Few left without telling anyone. But today we saw what warriors are made of.

I saw Dr. Pandya coming from the gates. He was a senior neurosurgeon and head of the department. He was old, but he was the first to come. When we all saw him coming, we felt a bit relieved. Neurosurgeon resident Dr. Modh"Sir, how are you? I hope everything is well at home. He shouted back, "Doctor, leave all that aside. Tell me what the situation is. And where is that superintendent of ours and other incharges?" I said, "Sir, we called him, but he said he was busy with his family's well-being. And till now, no senior consultant has been here. Few came for rounds, but when they saw this, they rushed back to their families.``

Dr. Pandya"Ok, leave all this. Let's gather all those present here. Come on, people, call everyone here.

There was a huge commotion everywhere. The pathway on the hospital campus was now chockablock, and so lines went on to the main road. Since vehicles could not come, people were rushing in with a limping gait, carrying their injured relatives on their backs or hands. The scene was very scary and depressing. We all shouted for all the fellow doctors and paramedics to gather in the OPD hall. When we saw each other, we were very relaxed. There were 200 odd people around. Resident doctors, nursing staff, ward boys, sanitization workers, a few from management, and also a few relatives who knew some medical knowledge Sir shouted loudly, "People, this is a huge disaster. I know you are all fearing for your lives and your families. But today is a calling from God, and He wants us to help our fellow citizens. So let's do that". The air of despair and fear was slowly transforming into an air of confidence and service. Senior surgical resident 'Sir, where should we put all these people who are coming in?"

Dr. Pandya" Let all those who are seriously injured go in the ward one by one. Let's first give them first aid."

One of the sisters shouted, "But sir, how do you decide what to give?

Sir "Sister, don't worry, we will have one resident in each ward. He will do a triage and treat the patient first who is more critical."

I said, "Sir, but where do I get all the things for treatment? You know, though we are a general hospital, we don't have anything to give. We do not have veinflow, vecoset, IV fluids, or any other injection in stock."

Sir looked really worried now. He had been in this hospital for 30 years, and he knew the situation of the medical staff. We only have a few basic medicines in tablet form. So he said, "One of you will go and call the store manager and superintendent. Ask them about the keys to the pharmacy room."

Two of them rushed to the opposite side of the road to do the call from the call center. They came back in 10 minutes. Since then, sir has sent ward boys and a few management guys to send patients to the wards on the ground floor. When they came back, they said, "Sir Superintendent has angrily said that he knows nothing about such medical stock. He said not to ring now as a few of his relatives are hurt and he is helping them."

The other fellow said, "The store in charge has no phone in his house, and so when we rang his neighbor, no one picked up."

He was visibly angry. He said to a ward boy, "Go and break the lock of the medical store. Take a few people with you and bring all the stock to Wards 1 and 2. Let's see what we have. Don't bring tablets as of now"

He then said, "Raghavji (our OPD incharge and senior most staff), please take a few staff with you out of the hospital to see if any medical store is open. If they are, then ask them to give all their stock of veinflow, vecoset, and IV fluid to us. We will pay them once the crisis is over". So now Navin and Raghavji took a few of the fellow ward boys to their destined place. Raghavji came after half an hour. He had a few boxes with him. He said, "Sirji, one of the stores, has given me this box. The rest of them are closed, as once the earthquake came, all of them panicked and rushed to their houses. We tried to call them, but only one has agreed to come back, and the rest have said no.``

By this time, Dr. Soni, another professor in neurosurgery, Dr. Tripathi, a professor in surgery, Dr. Mehta, a professor in the medical unit, and a few other senior professors have come with a sense of duty. There were also a few private consultants who came rushing to help their parent college.

Dr. Soni was like a Bheem; he said, "Raghavji, take a few well-built people with you and break the locks of all the chemist shops and bring all that is needed. We will deal with them after the crisis."

Dr. Tripathi" But brother, that will lead to a criminal case against all of us. We will be in trouble."

Dr. Pandya "Sir, if we don't do this, then many may die. We already have 10 patients in different operation theaters, and we need to start the operation as soon as possible. So I guess we will deal with the criminal case later on."

Raghavji got the zest of the discussion. He took 10 people with him a few sanitation workers and a few relatives. They went and broke all the pharmacies. There was a huge mob around to see what was happening. They thought that there was some looting going on. But Raghavji shouted back, and by then a police van had come. The police people at first also thought the same. So they came out with sticks and started shouting at the people who were breaking. But then they saw Raghavji. Since Raghavji has been in this hospital since its inception, he knows almost all the police staff of the nearby police station.

A police constable said," Raghav uncle, what are you doing? Why are all these people breaking the shops?"

Raghavji explained everything to him. He understood the situation, and despite law and order being his job, he knew today's disaster had to be dealt with first. So he agreed to help. Raghavji" Please help to control the crowd. And also help us carry things to the hospital. If you are around, no one will attack us".

The police constable, for the first time, helped them break into the shop, and then they helped them carry the required things to the hospital. The crowd, which was initially thinking this to be loot, went into silence and watched things unfold. They realized that something necessary and important had been done.

So now, with the help of senior professors, the hospital staff has become systematic. The emergency room, casualty room, OPD hall, and wards were jam-packed now. Beds, floor beds, and benches were used to accommodate all those who required help.

I reached the ward as I was a medicine resident and so needed to be in wards 1, 2, and 10. There was a huge crowd. I started my job. "Dr. Gupta, come here," Sister rushed toward me. There are a few patients here for whom we are not able to take veins. They are cold and in shock. I rushed to the bed. I tried to get a vein, but all was in vain. So I applied all the tricks I learned during my first year of rigorous training. I, with the help of other residents, did central vein insertion and intraosseous vascular access. We were successful in a few cases, but not in others. We asked the ward boys to shift them to the ICU. But the sister shouted, "Doctor, this is not a normal day. There is no vacancy in our ICU. The whole ICU is full, and even floors are occupied. So many have died there."

I was shocked to hear that, but then I realized the gravity. So we kept trying to provide the best possible care. We saved many that day, but we saw many lose their lives. Those who died were shifted to the opposite building hall.

It is almost 2 p.m. now.

Doctor, Do You Have A Family? You Seem To Be On Duty All The Time.

At one juncture, I suddenly remembered my family. It struck me like a bolt of light. I have not thought about them until now. I said to myself, how insensitive of me. Since 9 a.m., I have not given a thought about my parents, brother, or other near and dear ones.

I was now feeling fearful for them. My family lived in a high-rise building, and the earthquake was very terrible. I have heard that one of the buildings has completely crashed due to the earthquake. There was no news from them, as we had no other means of communication other than the local telephone. So I rushed to the central call center. But it had a very long line. Still, because I am part of the system here, I entered the cabin directly and asked the operator to dial the number I gave. He tried almost three times, but no one was picking. That was enough for me to panic. I rushed out. It was then that I saw Dr. Dr. Dalal coming towards me. I asked him about his day until now and also about his family. He was also very terrified about the same. So I asked, "Dr., let's go together on your scooter and try to find them. He agreed. So we both started towards our home. On the way, the scene was chaotic. There was a huge crowd everywhere, standing and sitting on the pavement. Vehicular traffic looked like bullock cart traffic. Everything was moving inch by inch. There was an atmosphere of chaos. At a few places, we even show looting going on. It took us almost an hour to reach Dr. Dalal's house, which would take hardly 15 minutes on regular days. When Dr. Dalal's mother saw him coming, she rushed out and said, "Son, I am so happy to see you. You are ok. Come in. Hey Gupta, how are you? "

Dr. Dalal's house was a bungalow, so there was no major issue with the building structure. Even all the other relatives who lived in the high rise have come over here, and there was in fact an environment of festivities there. The initial shock of the earthquake vanished once the family showed all relatives that they were safe. And once all were in the house, there was a lot of chit-chatting and gossiping. And when they saw Dr. Dalal, the joy was tremendous. I sat there for a while. By then, my stress had increased. I was also itching to find out about my family. I now realize the mistake of coming with Dr. Dalal. Now I was dependent on him. I should have taken my 2-wheeler and reached my house alone. But what was done was done.

I asked Dr. Dalal"Hey, if you want to stay at home, then you can. Let me take your vehicle and see my family". He agreed to the idea. So I took his scooter. It took me another half hour to reach my residence. We lived in a high-rise building. When I reached there, a huge crowd was sitting outside the gate of the building. There were 5 to 6 ambulances and 2 firefighters over there. My heart sank at the thought of some untoward event happening to my family. I rushed toward my block. I lived on the 5th floor, so I rushed up the stairs. All the flats were opened, and there was no one inside. Now I was more worried. When I reached my flat, it was closed. I rang, but no one opened. I banged, but in vain. Then an aunty from the top floor, Mrs. Banerjee, while going down, saw me and said, "Beta no one is there in the flat now. Your parents and brother also ran down when things shook. Your mother had, in fact, become unconscious when she saw things shaking. So they went down late. I don't know where they went. They might be in a nearby hospital or maybe somewhere else."

I was really worried. One thing gave me relief they were alive. Today, what I have seen has made me paranoid. So I rushed back down. I decided to go to the nearby flats where my uncle lived. When I reached there, there was an exodus of people moving out of the flat. They were carrying baggage and other things. I saw a known person, Mr. Bhatt" Uncle, have you seen my uncle, Mr. Gupta, and his family? He lived in H Block."

He said, "Oh yes. You are the one who is becoming a doctor. They have left the flat, and maybe they have shifted to the opposite party plot. I rushed to the Sakambha party plot. It was an open, big plot where every year there was a huge Garba festival in Navratri. There was a huge crowd there. They were all sitting on the floor; some occupied the chairs, and some were standing and chatting. I tried to find my uncle and his family. I walked frantically around and asked everything in between. Finally, I saw them, and I rushed towards them. I saw my father and mother there, and I shouted loudly

"Hey everyone. Finally, I found you. I have been roaming everywhere for half an hour. Mom, how are you? I heard you faint."

My father even this time said, "Oh, finally you've got time to search us. Since morning, you have not even thought about whether we are alive or not. You know your mother is diabetic, and still you did not bother." I saw him as if some alien was talking. I never thought he could be so impractical and illogical. I continued without replying to his bitterness.

"Mom, tell me, how are you? Where is my brother? Is he okay?" I continued without waiting for the reply "Uncle, how are you and others? I hope no one is injured."

My mother "Oh, finally I saw you. I am happy you are okay. Don't worry, I am okay. I have been telling your father and brother to go look for you. I was so worried for you. You are ok?"

I looked towards my father as if saying, "This is the difference between you and mom". But I let that pass too.

My father said, "So you would be sleeping when this earthquake came. Do you know what happened to us? How badly your mother got scared and became unconscious. It was good that your brother was there. He helped her. When all was running down, we both did not leave her there. We stayed back and waited until she became conscious. What's the use of a doctor in the house if he is not there to help in time?"

I lost my temper this time. So I said, "Just for your knowledge, I am doing my MD residency. Today is my emergency day. When the earthquake happened, I was also on the 4th floor. My colleagues and I have been saving as many lives as possible since then. We have shifted more than 40 patients to safety from different floors. We have seen more than 1,000 patients so far. So yes, it's good that you and your brother were there for mom. But then, if I were here, I would have also done the same thing. But I guess you will never understand."

I talked to all of them, and after I was satisfied, I asked my uncle, "Uncle, what will you do now? I guess going back to flat as of now will be mentally disturbing, and there is a high chance that there will be many more such earthquakes in the coming days."

Uncle" Yes. I guess tonight we will sleep here. We have arranged for our meals to be cooked here only. Tomorrow we will take our call and decide."

I then told all of them my decision" I will leave for the hospital. I am needed over there. There are a huge number of casualties and deaths. So

I can't be at home at present. I hope you will take care of yourself. If any need arises, then come directly to the hospital and search for me in the main building".

My father sarcastically said, "Oh, you are needed there! Why? You are the only one there. You should think of your family also."

I did not reply to him and said goodbye to my mom. I said to her, "Mom, please take care of you. Eat properly. Don't worry about me. I will be ok."

I left after saying goodbye to everyone. With a heavy heart and a sense of duty, I moved back to Dr. Dalal's house. I picked him up, and we went back to the hospital for a long night and maybe long days ahead.

When we reached the hospital, the chaos had increased. There were hoards of people in the hospital. There were groups standing in the garden of the hospital. Many were crying, many were shouting, and many were depressed. There was not a single face that had an iota of a smile on it. I overheard a few of them. One group was there, and a person was shouting, "What has God done to me? My whole house has fallen, and my family got stuck in the structure. After so many frantic calls, these fire brigade people came and helped me get them out. Now the doctor has come and told me that he will have to cut my wife's leg. Another doctor came and said that my son was in a coma. Why is God punishing me?"

Another person in a group was crying and saying, "The flats on Mansi Street have fallen like a palace on a matchstick. So many have died in that breakage. How can a builder be so careless while making such a weak structure? It is the only flat that has fallen in Ahmedabad. I lost my whole family to it. I could not even recognize my family. I was saved to see this day as I was out in the street to eat tobacco in a shop."

We reached the medical ward. The sister saw us and came running by, asking, "Where were you? We have been searching for you for 2 hours."

I said, "Sister, we went to see our family. Since morning, we have been busy helping people, but then we thought about our family. I live in a high rise, and so I was worried."

Sister"Arey, that's ok. At least you should have informed someone before leaving. We were worried. And I don't understand that once you have reached home, why did you come back?

I saw Dr. Dalal, and he said, "Sister, they are all okay." And remember, our needs are here. We can't stay at home and not do anything.

By now, news has come out that the epicenter was a small village near Bhachau in Kutch. There was news that lots of people had died there due to the collapse of the structure and were buried there. Huge numbers have lost their properties, one or more limbs, and their families.

Sister" Do you know there is news of a hospital in Kutch that has collapsed and killed 150 patients?" Hearing this almost gave me a sense of nausea. I felt like I would fall down. One of the doctors standing there said, "I heard from my relatives that in Bachau there is a huge devastation. It is a town of 25,000 people, and rescuers are trying to find as many as they can."

He continued" There was a morning parade of 300 girl students due to the 26th of January, and due to the earthquake, all of them were buried, and they died."

Almost everyone standing there felt the pain. A junior sister standing nearby fell unconscious. We were all in shock. I said, "These are just the initial reports. Once everything starts coming out, I believe this will prove to be the deadliest earthquake in India. I guess we have more work to do. Come on, people, let's get back to work."

The next 15 days were all nightmares, no sleep, and only work. There was no demarcation of the subject we were enrolled in. I and my medical residents assisted in huge numbers of surgeries when possible. We were part of the emergency team when needed. Surgical residents took rounds when needed. We all took turns to tag the dead bodies that came in. As the days passed, almost all the residents and professors joined and have not left throughout these 15 days. Many teams of doctors went to Kutch to work there from the city, and many of us were part of those teams. There were many doctors, staff, and other paramedics who lost their near and dear ones, lost their properties, and even had many relatives who were injured. But once the dust settled, they were back for the work because they knew that they were needed now. Our kitchen worked 24 hours a day to serve the needy and hospital staff. Sleep was a dream, but when we could, we had no place to sleep. Our hostel rooms were declared unsafe due to the frequent earthquakes that followed. So we slept on the ground outside the hostel in makeshift tents. These were chilly winter days.

In between, I went to meet my family. My uncle had shifted to his friend's house in a bungalow. And my parents and brother have shifted to a rental bungalow near his friend's house. They choose the bungalows as they will have less impact from the frequent aftershocks. In flats, even a minor shock caused panic. There were people who had jumped from floors because of these shocks. So then, after seeing them settled and safe, I worked peacefully.

The picture of havoc has now become clear. In a few minutes of the earthquake on January 26, thousands died, lakhs were injured, and more than a million were left homeless. In Bachau, the news was horrific. Out of the 25000 people, only 5000 were found by the rescuers. We doctors were worried about one more thing.

Dr. Singh, a senior orthopedic surgeon, was saying one day, "I fear the extent of disabilities that survivors would have suffered. And above all, because we doctors were working without proper and clean equipment, the disability and complications caused by such surgeries would be mammoth". And yes, he is right; when we have to choose life over suffering in the case of disasters, we learn to choose suffering. If we are alive, then suffering will be reduced. But we understood the meaning of well-built and advanced healthcare in the country. If only every healthcare center was equipped with basic equipment, a proper autoclave facility, and more manpower. Fire fighters, rescuers, citizens, police, the army, and NGOs worked day and night to get as many people as possible alive. But a lack of healthcare infrastructure would have definitely led to more mortality, more disability, and more complications. So maybe after the disaster, a disaster management program was started, but I guess the most important part was forgotten, and that is the upgradation of healthcare facilities.

Humans Are The Worst Enemies Of Humans. No One Can Challenge This.

Days passed, months passed, and I went through my punishment rotation because of my issues with the superintendent. But I guess we learn how to cope with all this and try to find some positive way out of it. So I studied and finished my projects during the rotation of cardiology at Shardaben Hospital. This hospital had only a 4-bed ICU. It actually was not a cardiac ICU, and frankly, the number of cardiac emergencies was also lower. So initially, it felt like an isolation jail for me. But then I thought, why waste this time? There is no one to disturb. There was no one to take rounds, and the irony was that there were hardly any patients who required rounds. So almost after 1 year and 9 months, I had free time. So I studied as if I had exams after this rotation. All that I saw practically during this 1 year and 9 months, I studied the theory of those subjects, diseases, and procedures.

So my second year in residency passed with a neurology, cardiology, and endocrinology rotation. The event of the earthquake has imparted a complete medical education to the residents.

So finally, the day came when I rejoined my parent unit as a senior resident. So as a third-year student, the work was drastically different. Now juniors were doing all the work. I was supposed to take rounds both times in the day and guide them. I had an emergency day when I was responsible for attending any emergency in the emergency room. I was supposed to attend the references from other units. At night, it was my duty to inform my professor about the patient's general condition. Apart from this, I started preparing for my final exams. But then, I guess God has his own plan. He wanted us residents of the 1999 batch to learn practically. We worked during floods and malaria endemics, then earthquakes, and now what came out of nowhere was dangerous and a complete horror.

It was February 27, 2002, and a Wednesday. Today was my unit's emergency. I had come to my house on Tuesday afternoon. It was a routine tendency for us residents to go home on a pre-emergency day. The work on that day, in most likelihood, was almost nil. So I returned to the hospital at around 830 a.m. I went to my wards, finished my rounds, and was waiting in the ward for professors to come for rounds. Suddenly a wardboy came rushing in the ward" Sister, sir, do you know what has happened in Godhra?"

Sister 'No, I don't know."

Ward boy "I just heard that a train bogie was set on fire and had killed almost 55 or more people. They were charred to death inside the compartment."

I shouted, "Hey Ramesh, why are you spreading misinformation? There is no such news in the newspaper."

Ramesh "Sir, I was standing with the police PCR van in the emergency room. They got the message that an incident had happened in Godhra and to be prepared for problems."

Now we were worried. Frankly, after so many disasters in Gujarat in the last two years, we wanted a peaceful year. But….

By afternoon, we all knew that a horrible incident had happened at Godhra railway station. Since 1990, India has seen many religious riots related to Ayodhya. The city of Ayodhya is attached to the emotions of millions of Hindus. The majority of Hindus have always dreamed of a grand temple of God Ram in Ayodhya. There is a direct train from Ahmedabad to Faizabad, the Sabarmati Express, which is a few kilometers from Ayodhya. Every month, thousands go to Ayodhya to pray and show their respect. It is a festival on the train or bus when such trips are arranged. So as usual, the Sabarmati Express was returning from Ayodhya, carrying pilgrims and karsevaks to Ahmedabad. Godhra is one of the stations in between. For unknown reasons, certain miscreants had lit compartment S6 and the other three compartments of the train on fire using inflammable liquids. This has led to the deaths of 59 people, including women and children.

Dr. V.D" What is this nonsense? How can someone commit such an act? Setting trains on fire, trapping people inside, and killing so many. What can one gain by doing such an act? This is terrorism."

Dr. Desai"Yes, you are right. And now this will create a huge divide in society."

I "Bro, divide or no divide, this should not start a riot in the state or city. Otherwise, it will be more dangerous than what has happened there".

Dr. Dalal"Yes, you are right. When such riots start, there are people who will instigate the public on both sides. This will only increase the suffering, killing, and destruction."

Let's hope better sense prevails. At least the incident should be investigated, and then the real culprit should be caught. By giving it a religious name, we may actually hurt our own citizens."

Dr. Dalal" Let's hope people remember last year's earthquake. Every Gujarati, be it of any religion, worked so hard to save every life, and since then they have been helping each other rebuild their lives. See how much Kutch and Bhuj are prospering due to such united efforts."

I" Yes, so rightly said. I remember how Hindus and Muslims made chains for help in our hospital. They were helping patients, providing them with basic things like food, medicines, money, and even helping hospital staff with food."

Dr. V.D" Let's pray things remain peaceful."

Dr. Dalal" It is so sad. So many have died due to such terrorist acts."

Dr. Bhagat" I heard that a religious organization has declared Bharat Bandh tomorrow. I hope that's only symbolic."

"Rather than a strike, they should have prioritized helping those who are hurt and also pacifying the relatives who have lost a near-dear one."

Dr. Ritesh" I live in a mixed community; there is a sense of fear growing inside all of us." Something is going to happen is the common feeling on the ground."

Dr. Dalal" Ya, my father came by today to meet me and give me my food tiffin. He said that after giving me the tiffin, he was going shopping. He will purchase all those things that are needed for at least a month. According to him, almost everyone in our society is hoarding things for bad times."

We could all sense what was going on outside the hospital. It was my emergency, but the incoming flow of patients has completely dried up. It was also a sign that there was an environment of fear, panic, and maybe anger outside. The day went by, and the train arrived at Ahmedabad Junction. There was a group of ward boys and sanitization workers going en masse out of the hospital. While I was returning from the emergency room, I saw them. I stopped one of them and asked what happened. He said, "Sir, we are all going to Kalupur Station. The train will be coming soon. Our brothers and sisters were killed mercilessly by terrorists. We will stand there in solidarity. It is time to unite."

I said, "But you all are on duty in the hospital. What will happen here if need arises?"

He shouted back, "Sir, my community needs me now out there. So we are all going to the station. If we don't stand now, then we will be wiped from here."

Another worker said, "How can they kill us who were traveling peacefully? We have not hurt anyone. There were innocent people in there."

This single sentence made me realize the gravity of the whole situation. I rushed back to my ward to take the rounds. I knew the coming days would be difficult.

That night, as I moved around from the emergency room to the ward, I could hear police sirens every now and then. I asked a police constable during a regular tea sip at midnight, "What's the scene outside in the city? The police patrol has increased exponentially."

He said, "Doctor, as of now, it is like silence before the tsunami. We are given orders to be on alert, and all leaves are canceled. What are you doing at 4 a.m. here?"

I replied, "Today is an emergency day, and so I just saw a patient in the emergency room. I was feeling tired and thought of sipping some hot tea."

I asked, "But I don't understand why the train was brought to Ahmedabad. By bringing dead bodies here, we will create a huge wave of violence and unrest."

He looked angrily at me, as if he wanted to convey, "Boss, mind your own business. When you don't know anything, why do you even speak? But he just said, "Doctor, it's the government's decision. Moreover, the maximum number of people who died were from Ahmedabad. And to prevent major tension, they were brought here. Already, there are riots in Godhra and Vadodara. And even the bodies were not taken to the Asarva civil hospital. That would have definitely created huge unrest. So the government took them to Sola Civil. And it was 3 a.m., so the crowd was smaller."

I asked, "Tomorrow is a big day. I hope things go smoothly tomorrow."

He said, "Frankly, there are cases of violence already seen at various places. Let's hope it ends early."

So, as a matter of fact, he also agreed that there would be problems for sure.

So came February 28, and then it all started. At first, it appeared as a few cases of violence here and there, but by March 1, the Army had done the flag march. And then all hell broke loose.

Lots Of Suffering And Lots Of Learning—A Better Doctor In Making

The emergency kept pouring into the hospital. The trauma team, orthopedic team, surgeons, plastic surgeons, and neurosurgeons became busy. Scores and scores of patients were there for this team. Rest all the residents became the unofficial team of this above specialty. The routine patients with fever, diarrhea, cold cough, cardiac emergencies, and other emergencies dried up. The casualty room and emergency room were all painted with red blood. There were sounds of pain, loud cries, and abuse all around. Though this was a time of grief and disaster, I and my other colleagues have understood that nothing can make us better doctors than a disaster(natural or man-made). We again took this disaster as the best chance to learn about trauma and burns. So for almost 2 months, we had extensive training in burns, critical care, spinal, and orthopedic/neurosurgical departments.

Dr. Dalal" Today there was a case of spinal injury due to a bullet. So I learned how to treat a patient in hypovolemic shock. The amount of fluid, types of fluid available, what should be observed, and all such things

Frankly, no books can teach us this. We can also see the response immediately. Even complications can be seen and managed only in front of us."

Dr. V.D" Today I was part of the neurosurgeon team. They were operating on the spine of a patient. He was shot in the back. He was brought to our hospital. So I, with the help of an emergency doctor, stabilized the patient. Fluids, antibiotics, and blood were given. The neurosurgical team was short on personnel as almost four operations were going on simultaneously. So I joined. It was thrilling."

Dr. Bhagat "Last night I was in the emergency room, and a few people with burns were brought here. There was a plastic surgeon, an emergency room doctor, a senior physician, and me. The patients were from different age groups. A child 14 years old, male and female of around 40 years, and an elderly person of 70 years. They had different percentages of burns. I learned for the first time how to decide the percentage of burns and the grade of burns. The fluid management is so different in such cases."

We were all hearing this with excitement.

He continued "The fluids given were all different to all of them. The rate was different. The formula was there to decide the rate. The elderly had many diseases, so other aspects were also considered. The first time I saw the use of injection albumin. The way things were monitored through the central line and urine output was also mind-blowing. Despite all efforts, we lost the female. The child is in the operating theater. The elderly patient is now on a ventilator."

During the course of these worst riots, the medical wards were full of surgical patients who were operated on and required medical care, as well as those who could not be operated upon. So daily for almost 2 months, we took rounds of surgical patients. The care the surgeon took while handling dressing materials, catheterization, and any dressing was of the utmost importance. The rounds of surgical residents were also different. More than the symptoms, the amount of fluid in the drain, urine output, fever, if any, and injury healing were talking points. The juniors were taught suturing techniques, dressing techniques, and how to prepare a patient for preoperative purposes. So in fact, this calamity and our working with the surgical colleagues increased our respect for them and their ways of practice.

The riots went unabated for two months. It took a huge toll on life and property. The same people who stood together to help during the earthquake were standing on opposite sides, itching to kill each other. In the hospital, we could also see the groups of people who came to help. Almost daily, there were ruckus on campus and protests against the police, the opposite community, and the government. The only talk we heard was of bullets, knives, guns, bombs, kakda, petrol bottles, gupti, arson, stabbing, murder, rape, and so on.

One morning, there was a ruckus in the casualty. A person was brought in with a knife stuck in his back. He was made to lie on his stomach. The doctor on duty came to take his history, examined him, and called the spine surgeon for immediate treatment. But the patient suddenly shouted, "I will not allow anyone to give me treatment from a different religion. He might kill me."

I lost my cool, and in fact, the whole emergency room went into shock and anger. The senior staff came, and with a police person standing nearby and relatives around, they shouted loudly

"Mister, how absurd your demand is. Do you know this hospital has 99.99 percent Hindu doctors, staff, and paramedics? For so many days, we have served every person. We have never seen what religion he or she practices. I have not come across any person in this hospital who has said that he or she will not treat a Hindu or Muslim. So shut up and let us do the needed treatment. And let me tell you, brother, don't worry, no one will hurt you over here."

I was really awestruck by the way the senior staff handled the situation. She scolded him and also pacified him. He was injured and was fighting for his life. There was huge mistrust everywhere, so his fear was justified. Throughout these two months, we saw scores of patients and relatives who were hostile and violent towards us and staff. But we learned how to handle this situation. Communication and hard, dedicated work help to pacify a lot of people.

Politics And Religion Are Winners, But Humanity Is A Big Loser. For Doctors, Later Is Important.

It was Wednesday, and it was my emergency. In the evening, I got a call from the casualty about an admission in my unit. I reached the casualty room. The patient was a young male who was drowsy and responded by opening his eyes. He had no movement of his hands or legs on the left side. He had a feeding tube in his nose and looked very weak. I asked for relatives, and his parents came forward. I asked them the whole story. What they told me shocked me. He was their son. When the riots were going on, one day they lost him. They went everywhere to search for him and even reported him to the police, but they could not find him. In between, he was found injured and unconscious on the road by police people, and he was taken to the civil hospital in the city. He was admitted there as an unknown patient. He was treated there. Since he was an unknown patient, as per norms, photos of such patients were published in local newspapers. If someone could recognize him, then it could help the patient. When the first such photos were published, no one came forward. The reason was that his scalp was shaved for treatment because he had a head injury. After a few days, when these pictures were again published, the father saw them and rushed to the civil hospital. When he found his son in this condition, he was broken. During the riots, it had become an unsaid rule that Hindus got admitted to Civil Hospital, Shardaben Hospital, and LG Hospital as they felt safe there, and Muslims got admitted to VS Hospital as they felt safe here. Though the majority of staff in all the hospitals were Hindus and none differentiated, this was what it was. So the father took forceful discharge by creating a ruckus and shifted him to VS Hospital.

I angrily asked the casualty officer about the reason for admitting this patient to my unit. This was a straightforward case of neurology and should have been admitted to that unit. But the casualty officer said, "Dr. Gupta, I know what you are saying is right. But I have gotten a call from our superintendent, Dr. Mukesh, that I should admit this patient only to your unit". I called my professor, Dr. DAM, about the situation. He said, "Yes, I have been informed that we have to admit this patient to our unit. So do that and ring me after all the reports". Once I got the consent of my professor, I felt relieved. I went back. I examined the patient. The patient has brought a single discharge page from the civil hospital that has all the reports on it. These riots and the type of patient have increased my kitty of investigations and differential diagnoses. So I went for blood reports and other radiology reports. I went for a sonography report of the neck vessels. I went along with the patient, and when the radiologist did the report, he said, "Dr., it looks like the vessel in the neck is completely blocked. You should go for CT angiography of the neck vessels."

I counseled the parents, and since the money was going to come from the government, we straight away went for the report. The report came in an hour, and it was sensational. It had pellets of bullets in the neck, and the artery was blocked. I immediately called my professor. He also rushed to the hospital and, after seeing the report, gave me a pat on the back. He then immediately called Dr. B.D. Shah. He was a dynamic and aggressive cardiothoracic and vascular surgeon. His surgical skills were very good. He was luckily in the hospital at that time. So he also came to the ward. We all examined the patient again and also saw the angiography report. Dr. B.D. Shah immediately said, "We need to operate and see how he responds". We all counseled the parents and also called the superintendent about the decision. Once all were on the same page, the patient was taken into surgery by 10 p.m. that night. I was excited to see such a case. So I got permission from Dr. B.D. Shah to remain in the operation theater. But frankly, the excitement was short-lived. The operation was nothing like I imagined. Sir and his team of operators all wore microscope eyeglasses and were operating through a small incision. I could not see anything. And since it was a complicated surgery, there was a pin-drop silence. So I was yawning in 15 minutes in surgery, and so finally I left even without informing the team. I went to the ward and slept.

The next morning, the first thing I did was run to the cardiac ICU to see the progress. The patient was there on ventilator support, and his notes said that Sir has opened the vessel and he is clinically stable.

As I saw the senior CT surgery resident, I approached him and asked about everything. He was irritated due to the late-night surgery. But he knew I was the person who had diagnosed this case, and so with respect, he told me, "It was complicated. Sir has tried to remove the pellets, but they were so critically placed that he thought they might get dislodged. Sir has opened the vessel by doing a thrombectomy. This will restart his blood supply to the brain. He will be removed from the ventilator by afternoon, and once we see recovery, we will shift him to your ward."

I felt goose bumps. I thought if healthcare can provide financial security and if doctors are ready to work anytime of the day without the fear of financial issues (both of their own and those of their patients), then this job is satisfactory. But then, a dream is a dream.

This patient was then shifted back to my ward, as said by the senior doctor. Our team took all care, and afterward, medicine and rehabilitation were done as per medical norms. He showed a steady recovery. He was conscious and responding to commands, though he could not speak. It was a month, and now the physiotherapist was confident that we can make him walk slowly with support. So they started that exercise also. The patient's father came one day and said, "Sir, it has been more than a month here and almost 2 months since this event. We want to go home. We don't know what has happened to our home. We also need to go to the government office for compensation. Please give us a discharge."

I could understand their mental state. We have seen them cry almost every day. He was their only son, and now they don't know what will happen to him. Their lives, home, and kids were all lost in a single event. Once he told me, "I don't know whom to curse. God has punished us for being obedient to him. I don't know those who have burned the train, but I curse them daily as no religion teaches such an act. I also want to curse the people who did this to my kid. They had hurt him, though he was not responsible for the train burning. I am sure those people were not the ones who lost their relatives in the burning train compartment." The mother never stopped crying. She was always staring at her son and then at the sky, as if asking God to forgive them for some misdeed.

I told my professor about the parents' wish to take a discharge. Dr. DAM then examined the patient and, after due diligence, agreed to discharge him. He advised on everything that was needed. He then said, "Dr., go and ask Dr. B.D. Shah about his advice and when he would like to see him in follow-up. Also inform the superintendent about the decision to discharge." He then gave me golden advice that helped me prevent a major problem in my future life. He said, Gupta, you also do a few more things. **Get a Xerox of all the papers for this patient. Also, get a Xerox** of all the papers he carried when he was shifted from the civil hospital. Recheck all the things in the case papers and write down all that is lacking. Take the signature of the parents writing that they wish to take discharge and that we have agreed to do so with parents responsibilities and consent."

I asked, "Sir, why do we require Xerox?"

He said, "This is a riot victim. The cases of riots can go on for years. At some point, we can be called as witnesses. At that juncture, we might not find any papers. Then it will be difficult to say anything without papers. Second, anyone can accuse us of negligence. At that point, paperwork will help us. No one cares how much pain we took to treat or what our differential diagnosis was."

I asked, "Sir, but in our profession, every symptom has so many reasons; we then evaluate them, and we then decide on the best possible diagnosis. But it's not necessary that we are right every time."

Sir" You are right. It's not as if we will be accused of negligence every time. But when someone does that, the court will rely only on papers. If it is written on case paper, you are right. Even if you thought about it while actually treating, and though you would have explained it to relatives on that day, nothing will matter. Only what is written is truth."

"But sir, this type of law is okay in western countries where the number of patients is limited. But here we see almost hundreds of patients daily, and above all, none of the papers are computerized. We give it all to the patient. They might keep the papers safe or throw them away. They don't even bring papers every time. So then how come we are only negligent?

Sir "The problem with the court of law is that they will never understand what we go through in day-to-day life. With rising cases, rising reports, and the increasing possibility of failure or unsuccessful treatment, as well as a rise in the cost of treatment, we will face such cases. So start understanding the importance of writing case papers properly."

I" I agree, sir. But many of my friends are in the USA, and they say because of this, the treatment suffers. Doctors are spending more time writing things and prescribing based on protocols, and no one is ready to take the risk of making tricky decisions to save lives. One thing they ask themselves is, "If this patient sues us, how will we defend ourselves?"

Sir "Yes, that's right. This is called defensive practice. Don't start treatment until you have a confirmed diagnosis. There is no place for clinical judgment now. Refer everything to the specialty and let them write on paper what investigation or treatment to give."

"How is this possible in India, sir? We have millions of patients. They are poor, and we can't wait for reports to confirm their diagnosis. Referring to specialties will increase the cost."

Sir" Doctor, this is a never-ending argument. But putting doctors in the consumer forum itself sets a deadly precedent. Questioning our way of practicing and thinking is impractical and illogical. But then the judiciary and policymakers work from different perspectives."

I knew sir was facing such things daily in his private practice. He revealed that even doctor associations are getting more applications for professional protection schemes. But since the day I joined this unit because of Dr. DAM, I have learned so many things that would help in private practice. From clinical to management to communication to even maintaining case papers, they are going to help me in my future career.

Time To Get The Final Degree. Hurray

In postgraduate studies, the third year is the most crucial year. This is the time when you start getting confidence regarding the majority of the diagnosis and treatment. You start seeing patients who respond to your treatment. You try to finesse your art of clinical judgment and communication. Luckily in third year I had 2 first year residents. So I gave my full attention to them. To teach them I was supposed to study. Their questions made me read more.

Along with this we start preparing for our final exams. The exams are the most stressful things in the life of a post graduate medical student. There are lots of factors that play in these exams. The question papers are tricky and there is no actual course from where the paper comes. The horizon is infinite. Then there are viva exams where oral examinations are taken on actual patients. The fate here is decided by 6 examiners. Their intelligence and their mood on that day plays a major factor. The other day someone commented" Do you know MBBS and post grade medical exams are the two maximum stressful examination in world."

I commented" Yes, rightly said. We see so many students taking propranolol before exams to ease their anxiety."

Dr. Dalal" But the worst part is a lot of them smoke cigarettes. They feel smoking can relax anxiety but in fact it makes you sick and addicted."

I" But Dr. Dalal worst is suicide. Last year only we heard of 2 student's committing suicide in Vadodara campus. I think every student should have a proper group to de-stress the exams."

As the exams approached the group of 8 residents became closer. We knew if we studied together, helped each other and communicated with each other than this exam was not going to create mental stress in us.

Dr. Dalal" Gupta today is your turn to teach all of us about gastroesophageal reflux. It is a full question. So be ready."

I said' Yes I am. Yesterday's topic of clinical examination in neuro was wonderful. We discussed so many potential viva questions. Now I am sure we all are ready for any tricky questions during exams."

Desai "Dr. Vats was more prepared. She asked so many out of the syllabus questions. I was really tense. I did not know the answer to any of her questions."

Dr. Dalal saw me and we laughed loudly. Desai was confused. He asked" Why are you both laughing? You are behaving as if you knew the answer to those questions."

Dr. Dalal" Desai she was asking all questions which are part of mental torcher type. We all know you get tensed easily. So she asked those questions which are completely rare. "

Desai" How dare she make fun of me?"

We all laughed as we saw some cuss words from his mouth which are actually rare for him.

Dr. Dalal" Desai tomorrow is a big cricket match between India and England. It is a final of the NatWest series. Let's watch together in Gupta's room."

Dr. V.D" What nonsense you are talking about. There is exam approaching and you want to waste time watching a cricket match.``

Bhagat" I will be watching the match at Pranjals house. There is big get together and we will have fun.".

Dr Vora "I don't know anything about cricket and so I will not be part of the group."

Desai" I will not be joining as it is Saturday and I will be going to my house for the weekend."

Dr Vats" It's Saturday and so I have programs for the weekend."

De. Ritesh" It is Saturday and it's my emergency and so I will be running from emergency and ward the whole day and night. I will be there for dinner but since I have no knowledge about cricket I will not be joining you people."

I and Dr. Dalal were left alone. But we knew there was only a TV in my room. So come Saturday there was Dr. Dalal, me, surgical resident colleague Dr. Goel, Dr. Aman and my juniors Dr.Vimal and Dr .Nikesh. So then we saw complete match.

It was a thrilling, high scoring match. We all enjoyed it a lot. We made so much noise that the warden came up and scolded us. But then he knew we were exam going students. He said" You all are going to give the exams. I know your mental stress. But your shouting is disturbing other students. So lower down the voice or else I will remove the TV from your room. As such, it is also illegal to keep TV in your room."

We assured him to be disciplined but what happened then was he himself sat in the room to see the final overs. The loud noise he made on every run and every four by Indian cricketers led to laughter all around. He said" How can I not shout? These two young boys are playing so superb. Kaif and Yuvraj are terrific. Look at their aggression. "

Dr. Dalal" One thing is very striking. They are young cricketers. The pressure is immense but the way they are playing, the joy they have at every run and the team work they are showing is tremendous."

I" Dr. Dalal we are doing the same with our exams. Teamwork and stress-free period. It will help us to give this exams without problem."

Dr. Dalal" Bro just shut up and see the match. What type of comparison are you making?"

India won the match. There were bursting firecrackers all around. We heard that resident doctors have broken chairs in the canteen tv room. In the boys hostel one of our colleagues got so excited that he broke the TV itself. We danced and sang loudly. The scene of Indian captain Saurav Ganguly removing his T-shirt and dancing was euphoric. His lip reading itself showed that he was speaking cuss words to many England players especially Flintoff. Flintoff did a shirtless running lap in Mumbai when they won against us. In Fact I can say with certainty that half of India was speaking one or another cuss word to Flintoff along with Saurav.

Our third year went on and time came when exams also were completed and we got our results also. We all and in fact all our fellow colleagues in every speciality passed with flying colors. We were all consultants now. So now after 10 years I have finally achieved my goal of being called Dr Gupta with a degree to flash.

After passing we finished our stipulated three years. Out of 8 of us, four of the friends decided to move to America and settle there. Rest 4 of us decided to enter into practice and start our career as Physicians.

Dr Vats shifted to Delhi, Dr Vora became Assistant professor in our hospital itself and Dr. V.D started his practice as his father was a senior physician in the town. So he had all the infrastructure available for doing the practice.

I thought of getting more experience in a few of the things. So I joined the hospital as senior registrar in cardiology. I had a crush on non-invasive cardiology. I wanted to learn 2d echocardiography, treadmill testing, holter and other non-invasive procedures. So I joined here for a year.

The year went by where I learnt a lot about cardiology and learnt everything possible in non- invasive cardiology procedure. Since I was confident of my skills, my senior colleagues also showed confidence in me. In those days many cardiologist use to visit different small cities to do regular OPD and perform echocardiography there itself. So they started sending me to various such center in place of them. This helped my confidence and by end of the registrar ship I was ready to plunge in the world of medical profession.

Oh Man. This Was Not In The Book. And This Is Just The Start

I finished my stint in the hospital and fortunately because of my work I immediately got a job offer in the corporate hospital of the town, ASHA hospital. It was the first corporate hospital of the state. It was near to my house and I joined the ICU as a registrar. The difference was visible and for everyone to feel. When I entered the hospital there was security all around. They asked me about my purpose for the visit. When I said I have joined here as a registrar they asked me to let them check my backpack. I was shocked. I have never seen anyone being stopped at the gate of the hospital. Why would anyone visit a hospital for just roaming purposes? And checking my bag was insulting. So when I asked back for the purpose of checking my bag? He said" We don't allow any food item inside. And on entry and exit both times the bag will be checked. We do this because there are possibilities of theft in the hospital."

I felt insulted and was very angry. First day and it appeared I was a slave. I did what he said. While I was doing this and going towards the ICU I remembered the discussion my professor Dr.DAM had with me.

Sir" Gupta you are going out to pursue your career in medicine. But remember there is a gross change in the time you entered in MBBS and now when you are entering into the arena of practice."

I was anxious" Sir I did not get you. Why is it different?"

He said" See when you entered in the MBBS the private practice involved having a nursing home and clinic. All Physicians did this type of practice. Few who could not afford then they join some trust hospital, semi government hospital or government hospital"

He continued" But just like Mumbai and Delhi, Gujarat is also moving towards corporate hospitals."

I asked" What is a corporate hospital? I have heard only about corporate houses."

He said" This are the hospitals that are made by businessmen, rich doctors or multiple doctors. This are run by people who have studied management courses. The only principle here will be profit and loss."

I was interested now" Sir but then that's ok. How will that affect us?"

He said" Tell me if a patient comes to a government hospital or a nursing home can he meet you directly?"

I said" Yes. In our profession patients directly meet us and we attend them directly."

He again asked" In your or any nursing home if the patient comes will you ask for money first. Will you ask for a deposit of money?"

I said" Till date I have never heard you saying this to your patient. I doubt we will do that. Normally they come and see us and then they pay while they go back"

He asked" In your OPD or nursing home who decides your fees and other charges?"

I said" Obviously sir it is me. Sometimes we have to reduce the charges also. Sometimes we don't charge either. Sometimes patient pay at a later date also. That's what you have said in this three years to us."

He again asked" Who will give appointments to your patient and will you refer all of them to the specialist?"

I said" I don't remember you or Dr. Modi doing that to your patients. You people always are there in your OPDs and whosoever comes you attend. Some ring beforehand and some walk in directly. And I have never seen you referring every patient to a super specialist."

He then said" In a corporate hospital all things will end. In between you and your patient there will be more than 5 people. A receptionist, a marketing personnel, a coordinator, a billing person, and then a management guy or administrator. Before your patient will reach you he will have to pass through securities and this people."

I shuddered at the thought" Sir but then how is it possible? A patient is the one who suffers and would like to meet a doctor as early as possible."

Sir" Exactly but now there will be management, different department personnel, insurance desk and army of lawyers waiting to sue you."

I" Seriously this will create a big rift and break the patient and doctor relationship."

Sir" We doctors have been included in the ambit of consumer protection act since 1994. Now the early days of it are over. Slowly and steadily people and lawyers are using this against doctors. With increasing cases the way you practice will change."

I" Sir now you are scaring me."

Sir" No, don't get scared. But prepare for it. If you are practicing the right medicine and taking care of a few things then it will not affect you."

Sir" So if possible learn a few things now. Join some distance learning courses in Hospital management and also medico legal courses. I am sure in the last three years in the unit you have learnt a few things which no one has."

I said" Yes sir. The case of senior staff, earthquake, riots, the case of that patient from the civil hospital during riots, the patient who died due to mistaken injections and many more have left a deep impact on me."

I said" I have learnt availability in time of emergency, proper paperwork, write frame of mind while treating the patient and proper communication will always help"

Dr. DAM" Always upgrade yourself, don't allow new methods to outshine the old tested methods of clinical practice, and learn new chapters to remain in sync with healthcare up gradation."

I thought" Sir, this is a whole new syllabus. But I guess it will help me only."

Sir laughed" You have just thought of entering into practice. **No books can teach you what you are going to learn in practice. Every patient will be a chapter which will be absent from the book. Observe and learn."**

I thought sir's advice were golden words.

Thinking this, I entered the ICU. It looked like a five star hotel. There were state of the art beds, monitors, ventilators, and other machines. The staff was well dressed and standing at each bed. The ward boys were there who looked attentive. Every patient data was maintained in a case sheet. I have never seen such things during residency.

Every patient's data was there in the file. The history was properly written, every detail was there in subsections of history that we learnt while presenting the case in exams.

Sister" Welcome doctor. Today is your first day. I hope you will like working with us over here."

I said" I don't know about enjoying it but one thing is for sure that I will have to change my books. I am already seeing a sea change in what we did in the government hospital and what is done here."

As I entered, the doctor who was there on duty gave me details of all the patients present in the ICU. The round was brief.

Dr Pavra" So you have joined here. Welcome. Along with me we have Dr Chhaya and Dr Dobariya. We will arrange duties tomorrow so that we can run smoothly. I and Dr Chhaya also have clinics outside and so you might have to adjust. I guess since you are fresh it will not be a problem. Above that if you do overtime you will earn more."

I" That's ok Sir. As of now I am completely free and so will not mind doing duty."

Dr Pavra seemed happy on hearing this.

"So Dr. Gupta there are 4 patients in the ICU. Our work is to observe them and write the findings 2 to 3 times in a day. If any issue arises in the existing patient don't do anything without asking the consultant. Only in the case of a life -threatening issue you intervene."

I said "Ok".

Dr Pavra" If there is new admission, take the history and write in the case paper. There will be a prescription note with the admission. Just follow the advice to the point. Inform the consultant."

So after giving me the brief detailing of existing patients and imparting me with some golden advice he went away.

I took the rounds of all 4 patients. One thing that I noticed was that out of 4 only 1 actually needed ICU care. Out of the other 3 only 1 needed admission in hospital. But then I guess that's a corporate hospital for me.

Just then a new admission came in. I was excited to get my first patient on duty. As the patient settled in his room I went in. I started taking history.

Just then the relatives came in and shouted" Who are you? Don't harass him. We have already given history in the emergency room. How many times do we have to say the same things? Call our doctor and start the treatment at earliest."

I was taken aback by such abuse. First day and first encounter with a corporate patient. I still asked basic questions' Sir I agree you have given the history to the emergency room doctor. I am a doctor in charge of the ICU. I require a few details to write in your file. This file is important."

He angrily agreed. I started writing the history in the sheet available in the file. The sister standing nearby observed this and said "Doctor you have to write this over here. She pointed me to the booklet. It was exhaustive. I turned all the pages and it was huge.

I kept asking many questions as the booklet demanded. Then the sister intervened' Sir don't ask everything. Just fill it as it is routine paperwork."

I asked for the prescription that their consultant has given. When I took the history, did the clinical examination and saw the ECG it appeared to be a non-cardiac issue. I counseled the relatives. I said" Sir don't worry. Looking at his history and ECG it appears to be a non cardiac issue. He will be well soon. Maybe once a consultant comes he may shift him to room also. He will not require ICU stay."

The moment words came out of my mouth there was pin drop silence at the desk. The staff looked towards each other. The relatives almost burst. He shouted" What are you telling? The doctor has told me that my brother is having Developing attack. And he will require urgent angiography."

I was now really confused and shocked.

The relatives then rang to his consultant. And he shouted at him." Doctor, why have you lied to us? The doctor here says it is not a heart issue. And that he may not require an ICU. We just came from your clinic and there you were telling that he will require immediate angiography otherwise he will have a bad heart attack. What is this?"

I don't know what the doctor said on the other end. But in hardly 15 minutes the consultant was there in the ICU. He at first examined the patient. He counseled the relatives in a separate chamber. When they came out the environment was really tense. The consultant came to me and said" Ok so you are the doctor in charge here. Where did you do your post-graduation?"

I was about to give my introduction but he shouted" Discharge this patient and write the diagnosis as Cardiac chest pain. Advice for admission and angiography given. Take the signature of this patient that they refuse."

And then he went away literally banging the door on his way out.

I obediently did what was told. I completed the file as said by my ICU ward sister. I wrote my findings. I wrote the medicine that the consultant has written in prescription. Then I wrote the discharge. The sister then came with a form and said" Take the DAMA signature also."

I asked what this DAMA is. She saw me as if I had landed from MARS. She said" Doctor, where have you come from? DAMA means discharge against medical advice. The relatives have to sign saying that they are taking discharge on their will and it is their responsibility if anything happens to the patient.

I was surprised by this form. We never did in a government hospital. Discharge means discharge. I asked" But how does that matter? If the patient is discharged then it is mutual."

She said" This is for saving our neck. This patient if detoriates at home or after leaving this hospital then the relatives cannot claim that we deliberately discharged the patient. They took him willingly and so it is their responsibility. Once the patient leaves the premise we have no responsibility."

I asked sarcastically" Suppose the patient is really critical. And the relatives took DAMA and while being taken to the ambulance deteriorates then what will we do."

Sister knew the sarcasm" Doctor, in that case if the relatives wish to readmit then the process of admission will be done again. If they don't want to then they can go anywhere they want."

I continued my questioning" Suppose the patient dies on the way?"

She said" If they bring the patient back to the emergency room then we will ask for a postmortem and declare the patient brought dead. If they refuse for a postmortem then we will not fill any papers and allow them to take the body without any certificates or death certificates."

I guess whatever I learnt in 3 years was good for getting a degree. But they failed to realize that after that all doctors will do practice also. And looks like they have missed so many things in the curriculum. The education goes on.

Just then the sister came. She asked" Doctor the blood pressure of the patients in room no 10 is dropping. I have rechecked but it is still 90/48 mm of Hg. What should I do?

I remembered the advice of Dr Pavra. So I asked the name of the consultant and rang him' He shouted for disturbing him in afternoon and said" Why are you there? Don't ring me for such a small thing. Start Nor adrenaline injection."

I said to sister" Sister add 2 ampuole of noradrenaline in 500ml Normal saline and start 20 microdrop per minute."

Sister" Sir have you really come from MARS. What type of order is this? I have never heard anything like this."

I was shocked. I doubted my MD residency. I have treated hundreds of ICU patients and managed low blood pressure with ease. And now I have being told that the order I gave was from MARS.

She just then took me to the room and pointed towards the machine near the patient. She said" Do you know what that is?

I said "Frankly in the morning I saw them. I was intrigued but because of all this chaos I forgot. But ya I don't know what they are."

She said" Doctor they are infusion pump. Maximum we can have 50ml saline in that machine. Now tell me what to do?"

I thought I will go in shock. I saw around for help. The senior staff who was watching all this came by. She said" Doctor do one thing. Ring to emergency doctor. He will help you to learn this."

I thought" It is just first day and I am already doubting my degree and education till date."

The day went by. I did overtime on very first day as Dr Chhaya rang to say that he will not be coming in afternoon. I happily said yes. At 8 pm my day got over. It was not exhaustive as far as patients were concerned. There were only 4 patients throughout the day. There was only one admission which was also discharged immediately. But it was revealing in many ways. It made me realize how unequipped I was for corporate hospital. On the way out I met my old friend Dr R.Shah. He was an ENT surgeon over here. He asked" How the day today was?"

I laughed and said" Bro during college days I may have learnt a lot of medical things. I always felt I am equipped to manage any patients. But today I felt I am not yet ready to work in present times. It was puzzling, revealing and exciting also."

He laughed" Don't worry, in weeks' time you will get used to it."

The Hospital Is Not The Only Educator; The Family Is Also. The Real Face Of Corporate Doctors

I reached home and ate my dinner. But it appeared the day was not over, and my learning was also not. At around 11 p.m., I was sleeping in my room when my mother came running. She screamed, "Beta, come fast; I don't know what has happened to your father. He was just reading his book, and suddenly he fell on the bed."

I ran. When I saw him, he looked lifeless. My training during the earthquake came in handy. I examined his pulse and breathing. I was sure that he had had a cardiac arrest. So immediately I called an ambulance and started giving chest compressions. In around a minute, his pulse came, and his breathing also started. My mother was continuously crying. She has already called my brother, who was working at the time in another city. I kept watching him. By then, the ambulance had arrived, and with all possible care, I took him to ASHA Hospital. He was immediately admitted to the same ICU where I had started my duty.

So on the first day, my father thought of visiting my workplace, but as a critical patient. It appeared as if he had decided to take my exam firsthand.

His reports came. Since I was working in the hospital, the dilemma was which cardiologist to call. Sister told me to call Dr. SMS, who was the head of the department. But my senior in medical residency was also attached here as a cardiologist. So I decided to call Dr. Brahmbhatt. He knew me and my family.

I said, "Bro, it looks like my father had a cardiac arrest. Luckily, I was there, and I could revive him with a timely cardiac massage. Please come and see him."

He bluntly told her, "Gupta, you are already there. What more am I going to do? I have just come home. I will definitely come in the morning.

I was angry and shocked. The person has changed 360 degrees since residency.

I called Dr. Raval. He advised a few more reports. He said that I should go for angiography and electrophysiology studies to manage

When I asked him if he would come and see now, Then he said, "Doctor, if you decide about angiography and EP study, then I will come immediately. But if you want a conservative treatment, then I guess the treatment as of now is perfect. I will come in the morning."

It appears that a corporate hospital means that if a patient is ready for a costly procedure, then the doctor is ready to come immediately. Otherwise, the doctor on duty was good enough.

I discussed this with my father. He was very clear that he did not want to undergo any invasive procedure. He said, "I will not go for angiography."

I argued" But what is the problem? It will help us know the real problem."

He said, "You don't know. You have just come from your studies. Once they take me for angiography, they will definitely put a stent inside my artery. It has happened to all my friends. They admit, then they do these reports, and then they come out and say your artery is severely blocked. If you don't do this stenting, you may die."

In the hospital where I studied, there were all kinds of facilities. I have seen all types of attacks. And I don't remember any of my professors coming out and scaring the patient. There were so many angiographies that came back normal.

So I argued, "But dad. This is not true. If there is a block, they will tell you. Otherwise, why would they do stenting in normal arteries? Your friends would have definitely suffered from artery blockage."

He said" No. There are so many people who were told that their angiography showed blockage. But when they went to another doctor, they were told that angiography was normal. This has been happening regularly in Baroda. Even in Ahmedabad, there are so many people who had no symptoms but were still advised angioplasty and bypass."

I knew the senior citizen group had already made up their mind about these procedures. He was always a headstrong person. He did not even trust his son. I told him I would be standing inside, so no one could cheat us in this report. Still, he said, "You have just passed. You have no knowledge of this procedure. They will put fear into you, and then you will agree to what they say. And also, you are working here, so you will not disagree with them."

I felt angry, but I knew he was sick, so I needed to keep him relaxed. So I gave up. I did not call any of the professors to come. I managed his condition myself, as per my experience. Luckily, his cardiac arrest was caused by low potassium levels. So I corrected it. The next day, all the consultants came, as if they were so concerned about my father. He did not reply to them. He kept sleeping with his eyes closed. So I have to lie to them "Sorry sir. He is tired, as he cannot sleep at night because of these issues. But he has decided not to go for angiography."

Dr. Brahmbhatt"Arey.This is not good. He should undergo angiography. Otherwise, he may suffer another episode. The next episode will be life-threatening".

Dr. Raval and Dr. Pandya also said the same. They went one step ahead "Doctor, every time God will not be kind. And every time, you may not be around. Who will save him then?"

My father opened his eyes. He had heard this. So he said, Beta, don't worry. My God will protect me. But I don't want to go through these procedures."

Dr. SMS" Gupta, this is not good. He is your father. And you are working in this hospital. You should convince him to allow angiography and electrophysiology. If in the first week such a procedure happens through your reference, you will have a good impression with management.

I was really shocked. I guess this is another example of the corporatization of healthcare. I still told him that my father had made up his mind. I will try to convince him.

They all went away as if they were least bothered by his condition. None of them took a look at his reports or his ECG.

My father remained in the hospital for 4 days, but since that day, no one has come to see him. They bypassed the room completely, telling me that you were there, so that's ok. But the shocking part was that the head of the department did write about his daily visit. He said, "Since you have a insurance, someone needs to see him officially. So I will have to write down the consulting fees daily. Otherwise, people will get suspicious."

On the day of discharge, the claim was rejected. The diagnosis that the consultant has put forth is syncope under investigation. When I asked about that, he said, "You say it is cardiac arrest, but it could be simple syncope. And since no reports like angiography were done, how do we say what the reason was? And so it is still under investigation."

I went to meet the Mediclaim desk people. This was a new department for me. In the government, there was no such department. Patients were admitted, and they paid according to their capacity. The majority of the things were free there. So I went and asked" I am Dr. Gupta, and I am a senior registrar in the ICU. My father was admitted here a few days ago and was discharged today. I have gotten a rejection letter of his mediation".

The lady sitting there after opening the folder of my father said, "This is because the diagnosis was syncope under investigation. And mediclaim people don't give money for admission for investigation". I was shocked. I again asked, "But then he is still in the hospital. Let me change the diagnosis as per their needs."

She said, "It's not possible now. Once the file has gone and they have rejected it, they will not accept the new diagnosis."

"But then, if you knew this could happen, you would have asked us to rectify it before sending them."

Now she got angry "Doctor, this is not my work. Your consultant should have thought about this. They all have been working here for 2 to 3 years and they know about this policy of mediation."

I felt the punch. "So why did they do so?"

I have no choice but to pay. I got the employee discount, but still, the chapter on Mediclaim was added to my list of things to learn.

I took him home, and luckily he was feeling well with whatever medicine I had given him. He immediately called his friends to come home. By evening, all were at home and talking loudly. He said, "These doctors are all profiteers. Did you know that no one came at night to see me? The next day, everyone came and wanted only one thing. Angiography. I refused. And see, nothing happened to me, and I am back as normal."

Mr. Soni" You are right. See what they did to me. My son got scared, and he allowed them to go for angiography. I had just mild chest pain. Then they came out and scared him more. Immediately, he placed a stent in my artery. I had nothing, and now I have a stent, and I have to take so many pills."

Mr. Pancholi" What are you telling Soni? You are lucky that you did not suffer a major attack. Your son took you promptly to the hospital and got your angioplasty done. Now you can have a smooth life."

Soni" What timely? It cost me 2 lakh rupees. Luckily, the bank paid otherwise, from where I would have brought the money."

Mr. Pancholi" Not all doctors are like that. I missed the bus in the initial days. When my doctor advised me to have an angiography five years ago, I did not agree. There were very few facilities, so I did not want to risk it. Then this news of Baroda started coming, and I was scared. Then I had a major attack. Then, when I got an angiography, all three of my arteries were blocked. I was then operated on by bypass surgery."

Mr. Soni" Yours is an exception. Look what happened in Guptaji! He is perfectly okay. He had no chest pain that day. His son says he had a cardiac arrest. Guptaji does not even remember the episode. Maybe his son was wrong".

I jumped into the conversation" Uncle I know you are old. But don't talk foolishly. I am an MD doctor. I have experience and know what cardiac arrest is and what syncope is. So don't blame me."

I shouted at my father" Dad, instead of praising me for timely chest compression, you are worried about those consultants. It is their job to advice on what is in the guidelines. But didn't they respect your choice?

My father" What timely chest compression! Your massage led to chest pain. This pain is still there. I just fell down because I felt weaker, and you just started pushing my chest. You would have killed me."

I really did not know where to jump. I just stepped out of my house. **But that helped me realize India's health illiteracy. My father was highly educated, a gold medalist in his post-graduation days, and the chief manager of a bank. And see how health-illiterate he was. For them, even the human body was like a television set.**

The next day, the superintendent called me to his office. Dr. Gadhvi" Dr. Gupta, in the first few days only you have shown signs of insubordination. What was the need for telling the patient about a non-cardiac diagnosis? The consultant is allowed to do what they feel is right. A non-cardiac chest pain diagnosis comes after you do an angiography and the arteries are normal. We have seen many patients who would have suffered a major attack after being discharged with non-cardiac chest pain just seeing the electrocardiography."

I said, "But sir, this is not the case. I said, Diagnosis can only be made after proper history, examination, and ECG."

He shouted now, "Doctor, you are here to serve the consultant. Don't use your brain. Just do what they tell you or write for you to do."

I knew I could do nothing about this. Then he reprimanded me for not getting an angiography of my father, "You are a doctor, you don't follow the guidelines, and then how will you convince your patient to do the same?

I said, "Sorry, sir. My father is headstrong. He has his own reason for not going for angiography. There were some incidents in Baroda that scared him. And then his friends also keep telling him that all cardiologists do such things. They scare the patients and do things that are not needed."

He again told me loudly, "Doctor, it looks like you have no hold in your house. This has become a fashion in society. Do doctors catch you by the neck and do angiography, angioplasty, or bypass surgery? They explain to you, take your consent, and then they do all this."

I knew I would fail to explain to him that **"explaining in the proper way and then taking consent is different from scaring and taking consent. But then, I guess learning continues.**

As the days went by, I started learning that patients don't ask for all this luxury. They want straight-forward answers, communication, and a proper orientation of treatment. Now that the treatment cost was rising and corporate hospitals had added a lot of heads in billing, patients were confused.

One day, a patient came with a bill. He said, "Doctor, they have charged infusion pumps in this bill. Then there is a service charge of Rs. 10,000 on the bill of Rs. 100,000. The anesthetist has charged for putting a viggo. How do you explain all this?"

I sent him to the billing department, as frankly, I shuddered at the thought of getting admitted to a corporate hospital.

Come On, People, Stand Up And Welcome Dr. Gupta. Will He Be Part Of The Rat Race? Only Time Will Tell.

By the end of three months, I had decided to quit the job and plunge into private practice. So I went to meet Dr. Gadhvi, our superintendent. He said, "Doctor, it is too early to start private practice. Even if you want to start, why don't you do like Dr. Pavra and Dr. Chhaya? As your practice grows, quit the job. Till then, earn a bit through this job."

I said, "Sir, frankly, my temperament is not helping. I can easily get into fights with consultants for not obeying them. Just the other day, you yelled at me for my fight with Dr. Sinha."

He said, "But that was wrong. You performed the endotracheal intubation of the patient without informing him. So it was natural for him to shout."

I said, "Sir, in case of an emergency, what is the use of calling the consultant? By that time, the oxygen level would have dropped critically. Then the same consultant would have shouted for not acting fast. But whatever, sir, I feel, I will be good if I practice on my own."

Dr. Gadhvi" Ok. I will not stop you if you start the practice. Then do one thing."

I asked "You remain in this hospital as a consultant physician. I will generate your consultant's code. You can admit here and also see patients of other specialties if they refer you."

My eyes had a glow. From registrar to consultant in three months was not a small feat. I readily agreed. He asked his receptionist to finish the formality. I was relieved of my duties, and I was given a consultant code. So now it's my turn to take rounds.

It looked like destiny had its own design for me. On the last day of my duty in the ICU, while walking out, I bumped into Dr. B.D. Shah and Dr. BR. Shah. Both were my professors at the government hospital. The first one, as you all know, was the cardiothoracic surgeon, and the other was the cardiologist who used to send me out for echocardiography. When they learned that I had resigned from the hospital and was thinking of starting my own practice, they proposed something that changed my life. Dr. B.D. Shah" BR, let's start something in partnership. Dr. Gupta, do you have any plans or are you still weighing all options?"

I said, "Sir, I am weighing all options. But I am clear about one thing. I want to invest in an echocardiography machine. I have seen that the demand is huge, and it will help me enter many areas."

The eyes of both of them lit like a 1000 megawatt. They show each other. Dr. B.D. Shah "Oh, that's perfect. In fact, that's a rarity. A physician, instead of starting a nursing home, is thinking of an echo machine. It is costly and may delay your plan for a nursing home."

I said, "Sir, looking at what is happening in Ahmedabad, I guess corporate hospitals are the future. The patients are also asking for all luxuries, even if that means some extra bucks."

Dr. B.D. Shah "Fine, then let's meet today or tomorrow and finalize our partnership."

I was excited by this prospect. Straightway I was getting into a team of two leading consultants as a partner. I went home and started writing my plans. I wrote down my finances.

All the things that happened then happened very quickly. The next day we three met. Dr. B.D. Shah had a big nursing home for his OPD and minor operations. The plan appeared simple. I and Dr. B.D. Shah will partner in the machine, and Dr. B.R. Shah will make sure that work comes to us. The place where I will start my consulting room is fixed. I was invited to join the nursing home of Dr. B.D. Shah. So in hardly a month's time, the machine came, and my career started.

Dr. B.D. Shah had a roaring practice. He was the leading CTVS in the state. So apart from medical patients, I also got bulk echocardiography reports. We also purchased a treadmill testing machine within 6 months. So the schedule became extra busy. Apart from this, Dr. B.D. Shah started involving me in his day-to-day surgical cases as a physician. So my consultant career also got a push at ASHA Hospital. I soon became the leading physician in the hospital.

Apart from this, we both started doing regular OPDs in various cities in Gujarat and Rajasthan. Every Saturday and Sunday, we both used to be out with our echo machine. It became a standout feature of our visits. People got free reports and consultations from doctors in Ahmedabad at their doorstep. This became a huge success. Now they were our routine patients. And so whenever there was an emergency in their family or with any of their relatives, they would come to us. So that way, OPD became jam-packed. We started going to other hospitals in the town as part of the CVTS team. In a span of 6 to 8 months, from one hospital, we had four hospitals to operate on. From 1 patient a day to 4 to 5 surgeries a day and from 100 odd echos a month to 1000 odd echos a month. So now I was at home only to sleep. My parents never show me on weekends. In fact, I got the name of the second wife of Dr. B.D. Shah from his own wife. She used to say, "Doctor, you will definitely lead to divorce between me and BD. He has no time for me since you joined him."

So now the routine was established. I took rounds in the morning in all the hospitals, then came to the nursing home. There, I see all my patients and of the team. I carry out echo and TMT where needed. If needed, I do counseling for patients before surgeries. Then preoperative assessments are done, and a date is given for the surgeries. In the case of emergencies, I was the first responder. And then on Saturday and Sunday, we both leave for the destination fixed for regular OPD. So in short, my work hours increased, my patient pool increased, my driving also increased, my outside food also increased, and so did my weight. But who was complaining?

A Jolt And Loss Of Money, But Lessons Learnt Helped To Survive.

One day we got a reference from the cardiologist at the hospital. He has referred a patient who needs cardiac bypass surgery. He was critically ill and in the ICU. So Dr. B.D. Shah evaluated him and found that he was a very high-risk patient. He definitely needed bypass surgery, but when we discussed it, we were not sure about the benefits. We were sure about the immediate risk and possibility of him deteriorating post-surgery. But the cardiologist has argued that if we don't do anything, with his bad heart pumping and all three arteries blocked, he will not survive. When we put all this in front of the two sons of the patient, they wanted a bypass.

Dr. B.D. Shah "See brothers. I understand you are duty-bound, son, but you should also realize the risk it poses. This can be a very long and costly fight."

This one word, cost," has become a routine affair in our day-to-day counseling. I have learned a simple communication rule. **Every patient should know about the finances involved and approximate day-to-day expenses.** I always quoted a few bucks more while giving a figure because I have learned the uncertainties of corporate hospital billings. Another thing I always told my patient was "You should go and ask for the latest bill daily from the billing desk. Add Rs. 10000 to that. This will be your bill to date over here. By doing so, a fair judgment is possible about the approximate expense that you will incur and whether you can afford it or not. Because of this, relatives never got a shock on the last day. And they were well prepared in advance to make practical decisions. Many times patients did ask for discounts, but I have understood one rule of corporate hospitals. **If discounts are given, they will be from doctor's fees, not hospital bills.**

So all risks were explained, and the team operated on the patient. His bypass was done. But then, as predicted, he became dependent on ventilator support. It became difficult for us to remove him from the machine. His heart, which was already weak, had led to weaker lungs.

Because of both of these organs being damaged, other organs were also deteriorating.

Son" Doctor, why is my father not coming out of the ventilator? His bypass is over, and Dr. B.D. Shah said it was successful. Then why is his heart not helping?"

So this is India; you might explain the critical nature of disease. You may say his heart is bad and his lung is bad, but at the end of an hour of counseling, almost 70 percent will ask, "So doctor, rest, all is well, I guess. It's only this much, I hope".

So before the operation, we took almost a day's counseling to explain the patient's situation, what can happen if we do surgery, and what the risks are involved. Even the cardiologist has explained what will happen if nothing is done. They have weighed all possibilities and have agreed to go for the surgery. And now here he is asking the same question, which was almost the daily routine for the next 40 days.

I kept counseling them daily. This is one thing I have learned from my residency days. Don't **think that the patient will know everything. If they ask you, the answer should be given.**

Son "Sir, I know you are working very hard. But please do something. He is on a machine and still can't breathe properly."

The next part of any prolonged ventilation was always a tube in the neck called a tracheostomy. It took me four days to help them understand the importance of this procedure.

I said' See. As of now, he cannot be kept completely conscious because of the tube in his throat. This tube connects him to the machine, which ultimately helps him breathe properly and provide necessary oxygen.

Son "Yes, sir, that we know. But then why do you want to remove this tube and put it in the neck?"

"It will hurt my father". Said the younger brother. I could see pain in his eyes. I put my hands on his shoulder and said, "Brother, I know it will give him pain. But that will be for a few minutes. And that too, he will be under sedatives. But see the larger picture."

The mother was also there. So she shouted, "What larger picture, doctor? My husband is not recovering, and you are constantly doing one or another procedure. I cannot see him suffer like this". So that was the end of day one. After this, both brothers did not hear anything. The next day again, the same session, this time I tried without the mother. I started again, and this time I showed them another patient" See. This patient is on a tracheostomy ventilator. Look, he is breathing just like your father through a machine. Can you see the difference?"

The elder one" No. He is still on a ventilator. What is the difference?"

I said, "See, there is no tube in the mouth. So the fear of him chewing the tube as he wakes up is nil."

The elder one" Oh yeah. You are right. But then, will this help him get off the ventilator?

I said, "These two topics are separate." He can be off the ventilator only once his lung improves and he has enough strength to maintain oxygen levels by himself. But till that happens, he needs to breathe properly so that his brain doesn't succumb."

The elder one said, "What are the chances for that to happen to my father?

I said, "That can happen tomorrow, or that may not happen for even 10 days."

He got upset "Then, doctor, let's wait for a few days. If he is off the ventilator, then we may not need this neck tube at all."

I kept arguing but failed. The next day, it was the same. They stopped the counseling in between for one or other reasons. The next day, something happened that changed their minds. In the afternoon, suddenly, the patient started gasping. His oxygen levels fell quickly, and his pulse and blood pressure also went haywire. The moment the anesthetist on duty saw this, he knew that there was a strong possibility of the mouth tube (endotracheal tube) being blocked. He immediately changed the tube. His diagnosis was perfect. The tube that he removed was completely chewed and blocked.

I called both brothers. I said, "See what happened because of his chewing the tube. This is what I have been telling you from day one."

The younger one" But is my father okay?"

I saw his face and said, "Yes, as of now, the crisis is averted because of the rapid thinking of the doctor on duty. The tube has been changed. But this has led to a problem."

They asked, "What problem?"

I said, "Since the tube was blocked for a while, his oxygen levels dropped. For changing the tube, he was again sedated and placed in a mild coma. So now his ventilator settings are back to what they were on the first day. We will know about the status of his brain once he wakes."

The elder one was scared "Please, doctor, do everything. Please save my father."

I said, "You can see we are doing everything that we can. But let me tell you again. We are not seeing the results that we would like to see. It is taking too long, and his organs are not responding to the medicine."

The elder one said, "Doctor, if you want, you can do the tracheostomy. I am okay with that. I will sign."

I saw him and his brother. I said,"That's ok. They will get consent. I will refer to the ENT surgeon for the same. He will assess the situation and do what is needed."

These things went on for many days. One day, he started having a fever. The fever was not good, as it led to a drop in blood pressure and a rise in pulse. The high pulse was detrimental to the weak heart. And so, even with the ventilator, his breathing was not good.

I said, "He is having a fever, and the fever is causing complications."

The elder one said, "But why is he having a fever? He is already on so many medicines".

I said, " Agreed, but then there are so many tubes in his body. There is a tracheostomy, central vein, feeding tube, catheter, and vein flow in hand. Then there is a surgical site. There is also a possibility of pneumonia. There is a possibility of bed sore infection also."

I explained to him about the reports we had sent. And also what changes we are making to medicines. But then I told him" But because of fever, his heart and lungs have further deteriorated. He is not maintaining enough oxygen, even with a ventilator. If this continues, then he will go into a coma and may succumb to his problems."

The mother" Our decision to go for surgery itself was wrong. Your doctors knew that this could happen. You should not have done the surgery. We are laymen; how can we know all this can happen?"

I knew this could happen. Almost every day we heard from colleagues how relatives put the blame on the doctors if something went wrong. But then that's natural, I guess. I pacified her.

The next few days show him deteriorating further. He was not maintaining consciousness. His blood pressure medicine increased to its maximum. I knew these were his final days. And I conveyed this almost in every meeting I had with the relatives. I answered almost every query of theirs. I was available for them continuously. I knew they needed that support. I have even asked Dr. B.D. Shah to visit daily so that they can know that the team is working very hard.

Then one morning, he succumbed to this infection. I declared him dead and pacified the relatives. I finished the formalities. While I left almost all, both brothers, the mothers, and the patient's brothers thanked me for the effort. The elder son hugged me and thanked me. I said, "Please be strong. Take care of your mother and brother. And while taking your father back, if any formalities are needed, do tell me. You have my number."

Again, they thanked me, and with a heavy heart, I left for my routine practice.

I took a bath and reached the clinic. It was a routine OPD day. By 11 a.m., I got a call from Dr. B.D. Shah" Dr. You will have to come to the hospital as fast as you can. The relatives of that patient have wreaked havoc on her. There is a crowd of 2000 or more, and they have destroyed the ground floor. They have beaten security guards also."

I was shocked" But why? When I left, they had actually thanked me. And the formalities were almost over. Then what happened?

He said, "I don't know. I was just entering into operation when I heard the commotion. When I inquired, I said what I told you. Since then, we have all been in the 8th floor management room."

I said, "But what are they saying? Have you met the relatives?"

He said, "No, I haven't met anyone. They have said they will meet only with management first. Till then, they will not move the dead body either.

I was taken aback. I said," But sir, if you are saying they are a 2000 or more crowd and they have beaten security people also, then how can I come and enter the premises? They will be violent with me also."

He said," I don't know about that. But management has asked me to call you. They will like to talk to you first before meeting the relatives.

I shouted on the phone, "But this is ridiculous, sir. They can talk to me on the phone as well. How can they risk my life?"

He said, "Doctor, I really don't know about that. As of now, we are all trapped on the 8th floor. So try to come."

I again asked him, "Sir, have they called the police? At least let the matter settle down. Let the crowd disperse. Then I can be there safely."

He said, "No, they are not going to call the police. The CEO feels that it will lead to bad publicity."

I don't know whom to curse the relatives, the CEO, or, for that matter, Dr. B.D. Shah.

So I sat there for almost 10 minutes, thinking about my next step. I started my vehicle toward the hospital. Throughout the way, I was planning for my safety. As I passed another hospital, I thought of a plan. I parked my car in the parking lot of this hospital. I then took a rickshaw. As I approached the hospital, I asked him not to stop until I said. I have briefed him about the condition. I saw a police vehicle parked nearby. But there were no police on the hospital premises. I asked him to take the rickshaw directly to the basement. This hospital has a separate entrance to the basement from the main road itself. It took us to OPD rooms and the canteen. So, as I have guessed, there was no crowd there. Only people who had been coming to this hospital for a long time could know about this passage. So the rickshaw reached the basement gate. I went directly to the lift, which took me to the 8th floor. I prayed that there was no crowd in the basement area near OPD or the canteen. And God helped me, as there was none from the patient's side.

As they all saw me, they were surprised.

Dr. B.D. Shah asked, "How did you come? Has the crowd gone? Have the police come?"

I said, "None of that have happened. I came through the basement."

I was angry and frustrated, so I did not dwell on the details of my adventure.

I went to the management room with sir. There was the CEO, Mr.Sharma, other managers, and the actual owner of the hospital, Mr. Patel. They asked me about the history. In fact, the CEO blamed me for this ruckus. He said, "You doctors don't know how to deal with serious patients. Now see what they have done to the hospital. Why did you not handle them properly during their stay?"

I saw Dr. B.D. Shah as if telling him, "Sir, please hold me or else I will kill this man."

He said, "Mr. Sharma, before blaming him or my team, I guess we should talk to relatives first. Let us find out why they are doing so and what their grievances are."

The owner intervened" You are right, sir. But there is a problem. The relatives are now supported by a local MLA. The relatives are saying they will meet only in his presence."

The CEO" But that is not allowed. This will not help us get the right picture. You know how politicians are. He will accuse us of many absurd things."

The owner said," But sir, it is not possible now to meet without the politician. And we need to do things fast, as I just got a call that every media outlet is showing these things as breaking news. We are getting very bad publicity."

The CEO gave an angry look to me and Dr. B.D. Shah and said, "All this is because of you people. We have so many sick patients and so many deaths, but none have damaged the property or name."

I got angry now "Sir, stop telling this. It is absurd. We have also treated hundreds of sick patients here. To date, no one has blamed us for negligence. Even with this patient, each one of the relatives personally thanked me when I went this morning after declaring him dead. So don't abuse us because you have the power to do so."

Dr. B.D. Shah knew about my temper. He knew I could go out of control some days. He also knew I was right. So he intervened, "Dr. Gupta, cool down. And CEO, sir, please don't accuse us. Let's talk to relatives first".

The relatives and the MLA came in. They walked as if they had done something great and were enjoying our helplessness. Despite creating huge destruction and violence, there was no sign of fear on their faces. I saw both brothers, and they saw me. Instantly, they looked down.

I asked the elder son, "What happened? Why have you committed so much violence? How can you beat someone?"

The MLA intervened" Who are you? How can you talk to him like this?"

I said angrily, "Why don't you ask him and his younger one about me?"

The elder one said, "Sir, but they have killed my father. How can they do so?"

I was really shocked to my core. I shot back, "How can you say so? Who have killed your father? After all the hard work we did, you are accusing us of murder.

He said, "No, no, sir. I am not blaming you or sir for the murder. But the hospital has killed my father."

Now it was the turn of the CEO, and he said, "How can a hospital kill your father? We are not doctors. We don't give you medicine. They do. We are just service providers."

The elder one said, "You people killed my father. My father was sick. He required medicines and machines. And you stopped all that for him, and so he died."

The CEO" How can you say we stopped medicines and machines?"

He shot back "Last night at 12 a.m., I got a call from your billing department. The person spoke very rudely. He said that your 1 lakh rupees are due. Come and pay that immediately, or else we will have to stop the treatment."

There was a pin-drop silence in the room. I could see the perspiration on the faces of the CEO and other managers. The room was chilled, but there was definitely perspiration on their faces. The owner also knew what had happened. I was sure if someone had cut all three of them with a knife, there would not have been a single drop of blood from that cut.

I heard that, and I don't know what happened to me. I said, "Ok, sir, I guess it has nothing to do with us."

I asked Dr. B.D. Shah" Sir, let's move to the other room. Let's sit with our team and eat some sandwiches. This issue is not of our making. We have a big CEO and managers here who can handle this situation".

On the way out, I thanked both brothers, as they had actually saved our lives. We sat in the next room until late in the evening as the negotiations went on and on. Finally, it was agreed that the hospital would pay back the patient's entire bill. After that, the crowd dispersed, and they took the dead body.

I said to sir later "Sir, this is so absurd that the hospital makes such a policy of ringing at midnight. And above all, it is a sin that the relatives let the dead body stay in the ICU, as they wanted back the money."

Sir said, "The corporate managers are like robots. A command has been fed to them, and then whatever happens, they will do what they are told."

He continued" And remember, mobs have no brains." The siblings of the patient became mobs, and so they forgot to respect their own father's dead body. Soon they will realize the mistake."

I said, "But I guess at least we were saved."

He laughed" Your communication skills are coming in handy. You took pains to talk daily to patients without getting angry. That helped."

I said, "One more thing also helped. Not a single time did I ask him to go to billing and pay his bills. I only told them to see their bill daily so that they knew their financial burden."

The issue was then reported by every media outlet. Almost everyone reported this as medical negligence. None has the journalistic virtue to investigate and report for the right reason. No police case was filed against the perpetrators, and in fact, the van I saw while coming was parked there till the next day as a watch. I never knew who they were protecting.

The managment paid the whole bill back, and the team was also asked to pay our fees. When I tried to fight back, I was told I would face repercussions. The CEO "Dr. Gupta, you should be a team player. And if you don't want to part with your fees, then we can initiate an inquiry. The media has already reported this as medical negligence."

I fired back "Oh, so the team player comes into play when you know it was a mistake from your side. If it were the other way around, you would have asked for the whole payment from us only. So it's a one-sided street, I guess."

The call from the billing department to the patient that led to the ruckus still continued. They did make one major change, though. Now they call at 9 a.m. Now they also call the consultant about the same.

There was no inquiry to find out who the person who rang that day was. So when I met Dr. B.D. Shah, I literally shouted, "Sir, it **looks like in a corporate hospital every manager is taught to say My Way or Highway."**

About a month after this incident, one day while I was eating out in the restaurant, I met both the brothers. They came to meet me and said, "Sir, how are you?"

I got angry seeing them and said, "Oh, you people. Your father should be happy to have you as his son. You made his body lie in the ICU for money."

The elder said, "Sir, we are really sorry. But what can we do? Sir, we are small-time chefs. For the treatment of my father, we took loans from people in the town and village. When he died, we were under a burden of 7.2 lakh rupees."

When he died, my uncle bought this MLA for us. He said, "Son, don't worry. I know your father has fought well. If you want your money back, then do as I tell you."

He then told us to revolt against the hospital. We were told to keep the body in the ICU. He then called all his followers. They were told to create ruckus. He told us to blame you, sir. But we said, "No, we will not do that. We have got this call, and we can give this as a reason."

The younger lad said, "We get such calls almost every third day. But we used to pay the next day itself."

I said, "But none of you told me about this."

The elder said, "Sir, we thought you were part of the hospital, and so you should know the policy."

I refuted this and told them that we are visiting doctors and are not part of this type of policy.

The elder then said something that shocked me. He said, "Sir, we did all this to get money so that we could finish our loans. But that MLA took away all the money, and now he is not even meeting us. He even threatened to beat us if we went again to ask for money. He says that he has to collect the crowd, manage the police, and also manage the media. It all costs."

I actually laughed at him" Now you cannot go to the police either. Neither can you go to the media".

I felt mixed feelings anger, frustration, sadistic joy, and irritation towards the system. But then, that's how it is.

It's Time To Do A Solo Practice. I Am Self-Employed Now, But I Am A Daily Wager.

As days, months, and years passed, I also grew as a clinician. I got married and then, in due course, became the father of two angels. Having them in my life made me more responsible. I stopped taking risks and started thinking about their finances and future. I stopped out-of-town visits as weekends were the only time I could be with them. After having them in my life, I realized the frustration of the wife of Dr. B.D. Shah. When I stopped visiting outside town, Sir also stopped. Then I told his wife, "Ma'am, I have divorced your husband. Now he is fully yours."

She laughed and said, "But now I have become used to weekends without him. He will disturb that schedule now."

I can see the sarcasm in her tone.

I eventually left the team and started my own clinic. I made the decision to remain available at one hospital. This helped me understand the system, and even my patients knew that I would be available only at this hospital. I have seen many doctors running in different hospitals. This actually compromised the treatment and disrupted the life of the doctor as well.

Dr. Maniyar"So, doctor, finally things are settling for you. You have established yourself as a consultant, a good family, a clinic, and now a house also."

I said, "Ya bro. Finally, life is showing me a way. Before marriage, I was alone, so time was never a factor. Since I came home only to sleep, nothing else mattered. After having a family, I felt I needed to change the schedule. I need to take the responsibility."

Dr. Maniyar" But why are you only practicing in a single hospital? You can go to so many."

I said, "I have realized a single hospital or clinic will help. I get used to the system, and the system gets used to me."

He said, "That's ok. But then become a full-time consultant. Why remain a visiting consultant? This way, you work like a daily wager. Someday, if you don't work, then you will not get money either."

I said, "That's the one way of seeing. But by becoming full-time, I become a slave to the system.

Dr. Maniyar" No, the picture is not as grim as they show. You will have freedom. There is nothing like slavery."

I said, "Ok, tell me, if I am full-time, will they not audit my work? Will there be no sheets made showing the number of patients in a year, amount earned, and expenditure?"

He said, "Yes that will be there".

I asked, "Is it not an open secret that the management will tell me to refer my patient to a particular specialist only?

He said, "Openly, no, they will not tell, but ya, in a hush-hush voice, they will."

I asked, "Will they not make me see patients as per their liking? I will be forced to admit patients who are company patients and treat them though they may not require it."

He said, "Now that is too much. But if any patient is willing to admit as he or she is paid by the company, then what is the harm in admitting?"

I asked, "Will they not change the brand of the medicine that I will write? You know we choose medicines that are cheap and effective."

He said, "But doctor, that's ok. Hospitals are businesses, so they have policies for purchasing medicine. So what's the harm if they change brands? They will not change the salt."

I said, "But do you know their policy is high MRP, low cost?

He asked, "Now what is that?"

I said, "They will purchase only those medicines that have a high MRP. Then they will have bulk purchases from the company if the company is ready to give them at a low cost."

He said, "But then it is their negotiating power."

I asked, "Isn't that power through us only? Now if they purchase in bulk, then who is going to prescribe so that the meds don't expire?"

He saw my face and understood the math.

I then asked, "Do we refer every patient to a specialist? . A patient with cough to a pulmonologist, with headache to a neurologist, with gastritis to a gastroenterologist, with chest pain to a cardiologist, or with a mild rise in creatinine to a nephrologist."

He said, "Why should a physician refer such cases? Then what is his use?"

I said, "Does this corporate hospital not do this? In the emergency department of hospitals, direct patients are referred as per their symptoms. So this is a super-specialized promoting structure."

He said, "But how will that affect you? You can admit your patient under you and refer as per your liking."

I said, "Don't you think one day when everything is full-time they will dictate this reference in the name of medico-legal protection?

He said, "Yes, that has already started in one or two big corporate giants in Ahmedabad. This is what they do in Delhi and Mumbai."

I asked, "I know you are getting bored, but just two questions. Are they not asking doctors to close their clinic outside and be present in the hospital full-time? Will this not break all the patient data I have?

He said, "But if you are full-time here, then what is the need for a clinic outside?

I said, "Do they guarantee they will not kick me out once my use is over and they get some junior at a lower salary? What will I do then?"

I then again asked, "Lastly, will they give me leave if my kid wants me home or I am needed to drop off or pick her up from school?

He laughed loudly. He said, "Bro, rest assured, all was ok, but I know the main reason for your not becoming full-time is this. Enjoying your life and family is also important."

There was a cutthroat competition. But above this, there was a sense of insecurity between doctors that has been present since the advent of corporate hospitals. The doctors liked this concept as, frankly, they got more money per visit; they were only supposed to give orders; they did not require to maintain a clinic or nursing home; there were personnel to take care of discharge, mediclaim, and other form filling; and above all, the corporate hospital had a marketing team that brought patients to them.

Now, in place of all this, what they asked appeared okay to them. A hospital wanted them to admit someone who may not require admission or procedure, write more investigations, prescribe high-cost medicines, and refer them to a super specialist, who in turn did the same thing. So they were okay with this vicious cycle.

Hypocrisy Of The Highest Nature—But Some Doctors Are Known For That.

There were many consultants who were professors at our government hospital. Since this was the first corporate hospital, this professor got direct entry because they were respected and they had the largest chunk of patients with them. So initially, I thought this would be a blessing in disguise. I am a resident under them, so knowing them would help me grow. But it looks like even I failed to read that too.

The insecurity was so high that for almost many years I was not allotted an OPD room despite having a high inflow of patients. They did not even allow me to have an emergency day, which was given to the highest grosser. There were a few professors who thought people like me were their competitors, like Dr. Jain. (Remember the neurologist.)

When I passed my MD in medicine, I wrote a few articles. I sent them to a local state journal for publication. Within a few months, I got confirmation that they would be published in the journal. One day, I got a call from the editor of the journal. He was a senior physician and, in fact, a senior professor at LG Hospital. Dr. Desai" Is this Dr. Gupta?" When I confirmed, he said, "Doctor, you are summoned to my office immediately today before 2 p.m."

When I asked what that was about, he said "This is regarding one of your articles that is to be published in the journal. There is a complaint of plagiarism against you."

I felt a shock, but he asked me to be there so as to discuss further. I went there as requested and met him. He asked me about the article. He asked, "From where have you written this article? Is this copied from some other article?"

I said, "No, sir, this is an article on Status Epiliepticus. This topic was taken up by my professor in residency, Dr. Joshi. I made a note of his article. And that's how I have written this article. In fact, I have taken his permission also."

Dr. Desai "Oh, I see. If it is a note from a lecture, then it is not a plagiarism issue. But Dr. Jain has complained about this. I guess you know him."

I was shocked to hear that. So I asked, "Sir, but I have not shown this article to him yet. How did he know before it was even published? And why would he make such a complaint? You will not find a single sentence anywhere in any journal or even on the internet."

Dr. Desai "Yes, I have already checked that. But I wanted to meet you in person. He is an eminent neurologist in town. So he has access to articles in journals for pre-publication reviews. He saw that a resident of the hospital was publishing an article in Neurology, and I guess his name was not there on the article. This should have miffed him."

I said, "But sir, I have not written even the names of my professors in the medical unit. This article was written after I left the residency. Even Dr. Joshi sir has said no to his name."

Dr. Desai" Let me call Dr. Joshi for confirmation so that we can end this inquiry.

I said okay. He called sir, and after talking to him, he was convinced by my explanation. But then he dropped the bomb.

He said, "See, doctor, I will have to show something to Dr.Jain. What I will do is publish this article of yours as scheduled so that it makes a statement to others. But we will blacklist you for 6 months, and we will withdraw all other articles of yours. You can resend them after 6 months."

I wanted to protest, but knowing Dr. Desai from residency, I knew he would not budge. I was happy that at least the article for which the plagiarism complaint was made will be published. I really felt frustrated by the situation. But that's how it is.

When I started practicing in a private hospital, I was fortunate again to meet Dr.Jain. He has spread his kingdom here as well. No one could enter his den without his consent. No other neurologist was allowed to settle here. Even I heard that he had forced the owner not to allow Dr. Joshi to practice here. He instantly disliked me. But then, slowly and steadily, I was getting used to this insecurity issue. For the first 5 to 6 years, I was part of the CVTS team of Dr. B.D. Shah, and so no one came in between. We have the numbers, so management was also silent. They definitely made sure that I didn't get OPD rooms, emergency days, or even hospital-direct patients. But then we ourselves were growing and were in no need of their favor. As our work grew, patients came directly to us out of goodwill, and other doctors also referred patients directly because of our work ethics.

My academics continued here as well. While treating one of the patients, Dr. B.D. Shah and Dr. Jaim came together. He was a patient of Dr. B.D. Shah, and he has referred him to me. Since the patient's relatives knew Dr. Jain, they asked us to refer to him also. So there he was. In this patient, we have used a rare medicine to save his life. It worked wonders. So since this was a rare medical event, I wrote an article. Since we three were involved out of courtesy and ethics, I also wrote their names in the article. I thought of sending the article to the same journal. I was no longer a blacklisted consultant. Dr. Jain met me in the emergency room the other day. I took his signature on the consent form for publication formalities. While signing, he said, "Dr. Gupta, can I suggest something to you? Why don't you write the address of my clinic in the corresponding address? And write down the name of my daughter as a co-author."

I looked at him with a strong urge to shout.

(Hitting would have put me in jail.) I said, "Sir, the corresponding address is the first author. Since I have written this article, I will use my clinic's address. And your daughter is not part of the team. How can I write her name?"

He said, "See, she is doing a residency in neurology at VS Hospital. Having as many articles as possible can help her career."

I said, "But sir, isn't that unethical? She is still studying and is not part of our hospital. How can I justify her being part of the team?

Then he used his Ace card See, doctor, if you want your address, that's ok with me. But if you write her name, then this article will be published instantly. No one will oppose it."

I saw the hidden threat. I asked Dr. B.D. Shah about the same. He, with a few cuss words, advised me to write her name. But then I told him my story of plagiarism. He laughed and said, "Fate has a cycle. It comes full circle here only. I can understand your anger. But drop it. These people will never have any ethics or morality."

And sir, you were so right. Even after agreeing to write her name, his attitude towards me did not change. He kept opposing me in every way in the hospital, both directly and indirectly. But then, who cared?

Managers Will Be Managers. A Life Lost And A Lesson Learned.

I had many patients who became families for me. I was consulted by them on everything. Whatever the disease, they will first come to me and then follow my advice. They went to the doctors I referred them to. If one member did so, then the whole family and their relatives also did so in many cases. One such family was the Bhambhani family. This family consisted of Uncle Aunty, their three daughters, and one son. Even one daughter-in-law's husband and son were my patients. Aunty was my patient for more than 4–5 years. She had many diseases, of which diabetes was causing a lot of problems. Uncle had a paralysis attack in front of me. Unfortunately he was an attendant during auntie's admission. That day, I did all the formalities like his son. As there was no one with them in the hospital, I filled out all the forms. So I was both their relative and their doctor. This attack led to permanent disabilities in the left hand and leg. But Uncle was stubborn, and he fought back.

One day, Aunty was admitted to the hospital for recurrent fever. It was due to a urinary infection. Since her diabetes was uncontrolled, her kidneys and nerves were causing problems. So in this admission, we have treated her urinary infection and referred her to a nephrologist for further planning. Dr. Parekh was a senior nephrologist. Even the family was happy with his approach. So finally, the day of discharge came. Dr. Parekh has advised an iron injection be given before discharge. So after morning rounds, it was scheduled. Since it was Sunday, I did not come for the evening rounds as my family went on some outings. This was informed to the daughter of Aunty, who was staying with her in the hospital. Uncle did not come this time to the hospital, as he was at his native place.

It was 7.20 a.m. in the morning on Monday. I got a call from uncle. His voice was low" Son, please go and see your aunty. She is in tremendous pain. And no one is attending her."

I was taken by surprise. No one from the hospital had informed me of such symptoms. I pacified him and asked, "Uncle, what happened? Where is the pain, and since when?"

He said, "She has had this pain in her hand since yesterday evening. Some injections were started, and after that, pain started. She has been shouting since then, but no doctor has come to see her. A staff member did come and go away, saying that it was nothing. Please go and see her."

Fortunately, I came in the morning to drop my daughter off at school. Her school was across the road from the hospital. So I dropped her off and went straight to the hospital. When I went to aunt's room, she was crying in pain. I saw her hand, and it was all swollen up. I could see redness over her hand, and her nails were turning bluish. I asked her daughter about the event. She said, "Sir, yesterday a red injection was started. I guess it was an iron injection. After the drip, she started shouting in pain. So I called the doctor. But the doctor did not come. Instead, after calling three times, the staff came. She saw that the drip was slow, so she massaged the site of the viggo. So the drip rate increased. Though her pain increased, she went away. When I called her back, they did the same massage and finished the drip."

"Then what happened?" I asked.

She said, "Once the drip got over, her hands started swelling up. Her pain became tremendous. I cannot see her like this. So I sent my brother to the doctor. But the doctor came and said this is pain from vein inflammation. They asked us to apply ice packs".

I have understood the whole event. For me, it was clear that the fluid with iron had not gone into the vein but into outside chambers. This has led to huge inflammation in structures. Because of the swelling, the blood vessels are now compressed. Soon she will go into a gangrenous stage.

I asked the doctor on duty to go for immediate sonography and arterial Doppler. I called Dr. Bhatia; he was the senior plastic surgeon in the hospital. He also came immediately. He also agreed to my assessment.

I was angry from inside, but I have learned to remain cool in a crisis situation. I wanted answers, but I guessed that was for later. Her reports came, and the diagnosis was confirmed. It was compartment syndrome due to extravasation of fluid and iron. Dr. Bhatia advised an immediate release of the pressure so that we could save the artery. So after extensive counseling with the relative, the operation was scheduled. Preparations were done. I was counseling the daughter and son. I said, "I know things have taken a bad turn. But rather than talking about how and why it happened, let's first deal with this crisis. Looking at her diabetes, kidney condition, and last history of heart problems, it will be a risky operation, but we need to do it otherwise it will lead to gangrene".

The daughter shouted, "But doctor, this is sheer negligence. My mother is fighting for her life when ideally she should be going home today."

I said, "I am also angry, but I want to fight this crisis first".

Dr. Bhatia "See, I am sorry this is happening to your mother. But please listen carefully to what I am going to say."

He said, "We will have to put various incisions on the skin and deep down so that we release the swelling. This will ideally suffice to treat compartment syndrome. But if the damage is extensive and if I see that we cannot save her hand, then maybe I will come out and ask for permission for amputation."

Hearing this, both brothers and sisters went into shock. They could not speak for a while. They cried. Then I intervened" Sir, what are the chances of that happening?"

Dr. Bhatia then said something that increased the anger of my siblings and myself. He said, "If we had seen her tomorrow itself, then maybe the chances of amputation were nil. But it is almost 12 hours until the event, and we all know iron is not a good chemical to extravasate. So the chances are there. But if we don't do it now, then the chances of that happening will be 100 percent in a few hours.

They both knew they had no choice. So they called all their nearest ones and gave consent.

The operation went longer than expected. We have already talked about Auntie's other comorbidities. I was actually worried about her heart and kidneys. I was not sure how they would react to such a sudden crisis and anesthesia. I actually prayed to God for her safety. The daughter told me, "Sir, we are very worried. I am not feeling good about this. Since you have also talked to my elder sister, she has also left Dubai to come here. You're asking her to come immediately is also not giving me a good feeling."

I said, "See, I know this is a very critical condition. But we will do all we can. And I wanted all of you here because I was also not feeling well. If all is well, then maybe she will recover faster. And your dad will also get support. He is all alone at your home in ABU."

She said, "I remember you always telling us that your mother is standing on the hilltop. Everything looks very beautiful from there. But a small push will throw her into a deep valley, which will be deadly for her. Today looks like this only."

I was taken aback by this statement. I tell this to all my patients who have comorbidities. I always want them to realize the need for a strong defense against a disease. Diarrhea, vomiting, and fever have led to so many complications in such patients.

Dr. Bhatia emerged from the operation theater after 4 hours of surgery. He looked depressed. He said, "Dr. Gupta. Sorry, but the tissues are very bad. I don't think I can salvage the hand. If we leave it like this, it will get septic and lead to mortality."

Along with the daughter and son, I also felt the punch in the abdomen. I did not want this to happen. But I knew what Dr. Bhatia said was true. Leaving necrotic tissue in the body will always lead to infection spreading in the body. So with a heavy heart and crying eyes, they agreed to an amputation. He did that in the next 2 hours, and by 9.30 p.m., the patient was out and was shifted to the ICU.

When the son saw her mother in this condition, he started shouting loudly, "I will not leave anyone here. They have made my mother suffer. How can a doctor and staff do this? We have been calling for help since evening, but no one had time to come and see her."

I tried pacifying him, but his anger came on me also" No doctor. It is also your fault. How can you admit my mother to such a hospital? They are so irresponsible. They have almost killed my mother. I will file a case against them."

I knew he was right in his anger. I again tried to pacify him. After surgery, Aunty was not showing any signs of recovery. Her pressure and pulse were haywire. Her urine has dropped considerably. So I referred her to Dr. Parekh. He came instantly and advised dialysis if reports came back bad or if urine remained low. This was again an indication of a constantly deteriorating condition. Her condition was constantly monitored in the ICU. I did not leave her bed during this time. I wanted her to stabilize first. Her blood pressure did not improve despite all the medicines. Her pulse started fluctuating. It was almost 11.40 p.m. Looking at her condition, I have started preparing both of them for the final outcome. My clinical knowledge over these many years has given me an instinct.

And my instinct was that Aunty might not survive this scare. Her pulse again went very high. She went into cardiac arrest. We tried to revive her by giving her a cardiac massage and defibrillation. All the medicines that we could give were given. But after almost half an hour of effort, we gave up. Her ECG came straight, and there was no life left. So with a heavy heart and moist eyes, I declared her dead to both of them present. And the moment I declared it, the door to the ICU opened. The eldest daughter, who has rushed from Dubai, has just arrived. She rushed from the airport with the hope of meeting her mother. But fate has its own scary ways. She could not meet her mother one last time. All hell broke loose. All three of them were crying like babies around their mother. I started preparing for the papers. I called the daughter for some signatures when Dr. Bhatia came. He again dropped a bomb" If only we had diagnosed it early, then the condition would have been different". I thanked Sir for his efforts and told him, "Sir, I will take care of the rest of the things. They were all angry with the outcome, and so they decided not to take the dead body home. Instead, they wanted to file a case against the hospital. I knew this was coming. I tried to explain to them that it would not help and would cause a lot of damage to people who had actually helped. But the anger was such that they just wanted a case to be filled. I kept arguing with them. One by one, I met all of them, but they were angry.

After almost 2 hours of discussion, there was no headway. So I called the deputy administrator, Dr. Mistry. He was a young lad but had all the features of a manager. So when I called him to rush here for help, he said, "Sir, what will I do there? If they want to file a case, let them. Let the police take the dead body. We will deal with this in the morning."

I literally shouted, "Do you know what you are saying? Do you even know what will happen then? Will they file this case and punish the real culprit? But since he was a junior administrator and had nothing to lose, he refused to come. He in fact absurdly suggested something 'Sir, all these cases are for money. If they want, we can give them some discounts."

I would have killed him if he were in front of me. I told him, "Doctor, they have no intention to get money or discounts. Do you know they have already paid the whole bill?"

Still, he did not budge and disconnected the phone. Now I knew I was all alone. Actually, at one point I also felt that letting them file the case would put the hospital management in jail. But then I remembered a few recent cases. These corporate hospitals have a battery of lawyers, and they have excused themselves from each and every case, saying that they are service providers and we are not accountable for the misdeeds of doctors. Since these were the early days of corporatization in this part of the country, the judge also agreed to this argument.

So I kept arguing with them. It was already 5 a.m. in the morning. So finally, I was tired. I called all of them into a single room. I asked them to call uncle, their father. I said I wanted to have one final discussion. So they agreed. I talked to Uncle "Uncle, I am really sorry about your loss. I can assure you that I did all that I could."

He said, "Son, I know you were there for her. I am thankful you reached within minutes of my calling you yesterday morning."

I said, "Uncle, I am also equally angry about the reason for this condition. And I also agree that the culprit should be punished. But filing a case will not help achieve that."

I continued "See, once we file a case, the police will take the body for postmortem. Then a case will be filed against me and the hospital. After a few months to a year, hospitals, with the help of big lawyers, will get cases against them dismissed. And finally, we will be fighting against each other. You know lawyers can easily prove that it was me who was negligent, as Aunty was admitted under me. Then in that case, my degree may go, and even there may be a criminal case against me."

All of them were listening. Uncle said, "No, I will not like that to happen."

I continued" Uncle, remember that in all this fight, the real culprits are the doctor on duty and the staff. They will never get any punishment. So if you think I have done anything wrong to Aunty, then definitely file a case. I will accept the punishment. But if you think I have done what a doctor can do, then please ask your daughter and son to take the body home and carry the cremation."

He asked me to hand over the phone to his eldest daughter. He said, "Beta, remember, I am also angry. But nothing should happen to Dr. Gupta. He has been rock solid for us. He has done everything he can. So do what he tells you and bring back your mother to me."

After the phone call, the daughter asked me, "So how will we punish the real culprit?" I said, "What I suggest is that you write a letter to the management. Ask them to punish the real culprit within 72 hours. If the hospital does not call you for a meeting at this time, you can file a case later on. In that scenario, your lawyer can frame charges as per his liking."

She agreed to this, and they wrote a letter. I called Dr. Mistry to come as early as possible. When he refused, I called the CEO and briefed him about the situation. I literally shouted at him at the end and said, "Since the last 5 hours, I have been here facing the relatives, and not a single medical administrator is ready to come. Is this the way we handle such a crisis?"

He asked me to wait for a minute. He called me again, telling me that Dr. Mistry was coming immediately. When he arrived, all three pounded on him like wounded tigers. He may have then realized the real situation. He took the letter from them, assuring them that he would put this on the table for his seniors. Finally, the ambulance came, and they all left with their mother. I felt really sorry for uncle and the family. I did not feel relieved, despite the case not being filed. I felt a gush of anger, and for the first time on the way home, I cried. Uncle and Aunty always bought sweets, honey, and chocolate for me and my family. They always called me for chitchat. Their family was also very cordial with me all throughout. I felt like I had lost a loved one.

The next three days passed, but no one from the hospital called to inquire about and discuss the letter. When I asked Dr. Mistry, he said, "I have already put the letter on the desk of Chief Medical Administrator Dr. Khatri. I don't know what happened then."

I called Dr. Khatri 'Oh, sorry. I got busy with some work. I will definitely look into it in a day or two."

I said, "Dr. Khatri, please look into it now. The deadline is this evening. We need to call them today to come and meet us tomorrow or whenever they are ready."

He shouted back, "Dr. Gupta, don't teach me. I have much more important work. And what is there to reply to? They have taken the body, and they want to meet us for what? Do they want the money back?"

I knew this was a standard reply from a high-headed manager. So I rushed to the cabin of COO Dr. Taulolikar. I have met him once or twice, but since it was urgent, I needed to meet him. I went into his cabin and asked for some time to discuss a matter. He said" Dr. I was just leaving for home. Can we do this tomorrow?"

I said, "Sir, this cannot wait for tomorrow."

He was all ears for me. I narrated the whole incident. He knew this was serious. He was angry with the type of response the managerial people have given so far. He called Dr. Khatri and asked him to immediately come to his office. When Dr. Khatri told him he was leaving for his house and he would come tomorrow, Dr. Taulolikar shouted, "Dr., may be tomorrow you may not have a job here.``

He rushed back. On being asked about the case and the reply, he was completely unaware, as he had not gone through the file, the letter that relatives gave, or asked Dr. Mistry about that night's event. So I briefed him also. He then said the same thing that he told me "Sir, I am sure they want the money back. These relatives are the same everywhere."

I shouted back this time, "Dr. Khatri, why are you acting so absurd? Let me tell you, this whole family has the strength to buy such three hospitals."

Dr. Taulolikar pacified me and said, "Dr. Khatri, this is really shameful that no one went to help the doctor. Do you people even know how much it would have cost us? And above all, a patient died due to the apathy of our staff, and we did not bother to inquire, punish, or rectify the matter."

He then asked me to call the relatives. He said he would personally talk to them. So I called the eldest sister and put the phone on speaker. She picked me up and shouted at me, "Dr. Not a single call has come yet. It looks like the hospital has no conscience. We are thinking of coming tomorrow and filing a case against them."

I introduced both of them to her. Then Dr. Taulolikar said, "Madam, I am extremely sorry for your loss. What I have gathered from Dr. Gupta I am sure this requires a thorough inquiry and punishment for those who are responsible. I invite you to come any day you wish. We will do this inquiry in front of you."

She said, "We would like to come tomorrow itself. We are all so angry that we need a logical end to this chapter. We could not even do our rituals with a peaceful mind. Every moment we see only our mother's sufferings."

We all agreed on tomorrow's meeting. I then moved back home.

The next day, as scheduled, the meeting happened. Both the daughters and their husbands came. We sat in the auditorium. We went through the whole case in front of them. The daughter who was here also put her facts forward. One by one, we called all the doctors and staff that day. Finally, it boiled down to one duty doctor and a staff. When it became clear that they did not perform their duties, the sisters' anger took over. The eldest sister shouted at the doctor on duty. She said, "Doctor, you are a blot on the medical profession. You sat there at the console and did your gossip. My sister came 4 to 5 times; you had no morals to get up from your seat and see my mother."

He kept saying sorry. But the sister was in no mood to forget. She continued" Dr. Your apology is of no use. I can see in your face that there is no grief or real apology. I am sure you will move out of here and do the same with another patient. I am sure you will keep eating your food even after killing patients."

She even blasted the staff, but she knew that the staff would ultimately become a scapegoat. Dr. Khatri intervened" Madam, I will assure you that they will be removed from our hospital with immediate effect."

She shouted, "I don't want only that; in fact, put a red mark on their CV so that they don't get a job anywhere."

Dr. Khatri said, "Madam, please forgive him. We have seen that when we are very strict, they may commit suicide."

This actually took her anger to the next level. She said, "Dr., if he wants to commit suicide, then be my guest. Such doctors should do so before they kill any other patient."

I intervened. I pacified her. I said, "I think this is settled now that these two will be removed from here and a red marking will be put on their CV".

They were asked to leave and wait outside. Then I asked all of them" What else would you like us to do so that we can express our sincere apology for your loss?

Dr. Taulolikar said, "Madam, we can offer a prayer meeting.'

She said, "We have planned one. It is our private function, and we will not allow any strangers there."

I then suggested a few things" We can offer this. You can refer one patient every year to us, and we will provide complete treatment for free. Or we can provide education to one poor student in your mother's name."

To both, they refused. They said we have enough power to pay for such things. Then I asked, "Then can I offer one last suggestion? Let us do a camp in your hometown on your mother's birthday."

They saw each other and thought this was a proper thing to do. So they agreed. When they agreed, both Dr. Taulolikar and Dr. Khatri could not believe their ears. How can any relatives be so gracious?

So after apologies once again, the meeting was adjourned. We planned a meeting with their father on Abu Road to decide about the camp.

When I, Dr. Khatri, and Dr. Parekh went to meet him after 10 days in his home town, Dr. Khatri saw what these people were made of. The moment we entered the house, Uncle came to the door to greet us. They expected an angry old man who would not even allow them into their house. But Uncle said, "Thank you for coming."

Dr. Khatria asked for forgiveness, but Uncle said, "No sir, don't say that. It's God's will. And we are lucky to have Dr. Gupta on our side. We respect him a lot, and my wife treated him like her son."

The lunch was lavish, and Uncle himself served us with love. Then we discussed the camp. He said, "Dr. Gupta, it was a good idea to do a medical camp on her birthday. Thank you for suggesting this. This way, I will have a chance to host you again."

Then he took us on a tour of his house. From there, he took us on a trip to a tribal area on the back side. It housed 200 tribal people who were fed by uncle and family. They made many beautiful handcrafted things that were sold, and the money was used for their well-being. Then we went to the school, which has 30 or so tribal students. This school was financed by uncle and his family. Looking at all this, we were all awestruck. I have also come before to Uncle's farm, but he never showed me this.

On the way back, Dr. Khatri only said one thing" Dr. Gupta I am really sorry. I misunderstood them and you. We should have been forthcoming when the issue arose. Please make sure that whenever any member of this family comes to our hospital, you inform me. I will always come and greet them."

Did the managers change after this? - NO. Was this a learning experience for me? Yes. What was the learning? **Attend, communicate, and be vigilant. Since then, I have been asking all the staff about Viggo and to see for extravasation.**

Without Good Friends, Life Is Depressing. In This Medical Profession They Keep You Sane.

My journey went on, and every day I learned something new. For almost 14 years, I ran a single clinic and hospital practice. I was part of the ASHA hospital for almost 14 years. I was not a full-time consultant, so I was allowed to practice anywhere. But unlike others, I did not. I continued here as a visiting consultant. During this time, I grew from a team member of CVTS Group to an independent junior consultant and a senior consultant. In this journey, I came across a few doctors who became integral parts of my life. Dr. Desai is a gynecologist; Dr. R. Shah is an orthopaedician; and Dr. U. Shah is an ophthalmologist. Dr. Desai was a college friend of mine. So we have seen each other grow since MBBS day. He, like me, has been part of this hospital since the start of his career. When he joined, there was no space for his department. In these 14 years, he would have been shifted many times to different floors and corners, but he remained stubborn. We had one thing in common.

One day we were sitting in the doctor's lounge with other doctors. While discussing our MBBS days, Dr. Desai said, "I wanted to become a surgeon, and so after MBBS I went for the interview. But just before entering the cabin, I changed my mind to take ObGyn". He thought it would be just 3 years, and then no super specialization would be required". He continued "In our city, we had two major hospital setups, as we all know. Civil Hospital was considered a terror house for VS Hospital students. We feared the civil hospital environment. And during the time of the MBBS exam, I have seen a senior doctor, Dr. Limbaji. He gave me shivers."

Almost everyone who passed during that era laughed. Dr. Limbaji belonged to the B-block hostel of Civil Hospital. He ruled the hospital as he was very aggressive and politically strong. So the majority feared him. So Dr. Desai continued" So I did not want to go to the civil hospital. When I had to decide on V.S. Hospital, luckily an extra seat opened in my professor's unit, Dr. Raval. He was a God-sent doctor, a very genuine operator, and a great teacher. So I happily chose his unit."

He then said, "But I feared Dr. Limbaji, and I got into a unit that had a lady Limbaji. She had a history of slapping three previous residents."

We all laughed, and then Dr. Modh said, "But then we heard you went along well with her. We all knew it was boyish banter".

Then I said, "Dr. Desai, we have almost the same story. I wanted to take orthopedics. While standing out in the queue, I thought if I went to orthopedics, my life would be full of late-night work. I am a lazy person and have a high chance of having high blood pressure due to my family history. So after giving it a thought for 10 minutes, I changed my postgraduate subject to internal medicine."

Almost everybody laughed. Dr. K.Patel said, "Why are you bluffing? Who changes from orthopedic to physician?

Dr. Modh" And people see how much time he gave to decide about such a big change 10 minutes"

Dr. Desai" We had months to decide this, and you decided such a big thing in 10 minutes. Do you belong to Mars?"

I said, "Wow, you can decide to change in a minute, and my 10 minutes look shorter to you. Believe it or not, it's your prerogative. But, Dr. Desai, don't you remember that my merit number was 7th at that time? And you can ask Dr. Agarwal, who went to the best orthopedic unit in the civil hospital. He was next to me, and he got that unit because I did not choose it".

Dr. Desai "Yeah, I know that. But baba, why are you always with a sword? Why attack like this?"

I asked" But Dr. Desai I don't know whether you regret your choice of OB/GYN or not. But it only helped us. My two daughters were born under your guidance".

He said, "I have not regretted this decision at any point. I enjoy my job, and it is satisfactory. So many new lives come into this world. So many blessings".

I said, "But I thought you would have regretted it, as for almost 10 years this hospital never gave importance to this branch. Your OPD was in almost every corner of this hospital. Wherever they found unused space, they placed your table there."

He said" Yes. But then I persisted. I have purchased my clinic with Operation Theater in partnership, but somehow I wanted to develop this branch. And for that, I required support from the corporate structure."

I said, "And see what your persistence and hard work have done. You are considered one of the best high-risk gynecologists."

The moment I said those words, there was huge laughter all around. I realized my mistake quickly when I saw Dr. Desai's face. I said sorry and said, "Baba, I mean, in high-risk gynecology cases, you are considered the safest surgeon. People are referred from faraway places, such as Gujarat and even Rajasthan. Even big-shot doctors like you should be their doctor if they have any such cases."

Almost everyone accepted that.. Dr. Desai" That can happen only if it is done my way. Otherwise, if I kept my sword sharpened and removed it from scabbard every now and then like you, I would have been just like a general gynecologist. Delivery, cesarean, and hysterectomy would have been my fate."

I said, "Boss, I am praising you, and you are saying bad things about me."

He said, "See, if I want to excel in my career and if the things that are needed are infrastructure, management support, marketing support, and security, then what is wrong if we work with the management?

I said, "I am ok with what you are saying. But what is this about swords and all?"

He said, "See Dr. You keep fighting with the management over every little thing. If your patient suffers a bit, you fight. If there is an issue with billing, you fight. Just the other day, what you did was very bad."

I said, "If you are talking about my shifting four patients from here to another hospital, then what was wrong with that?"

He said, "Why did you do that?"

I said, "See, those four patients were from road traffic accidents. They came from faraway places called Halvad. They came to this hospital because they knew me and wanted to be under my care."

I said, "When this patient reached the emergency room as per the protocol, I admitted them under my name. I then referred the patients to orthopedics, a plastic surgeon, and a vascular surgeon."

He said, "That's perfectly according to the protocol."

But then, in an hour's time, I got a call from the emergency room saying, "Sir, the Deputy Administrator, Dr. Milind, has refused to admit under you. He says that they can be admitted only under an orthopedic or vascular surgeon".

I called him and asked for clarification. He said, "Sir, these patients are from road traffic accidents and medico-legal cases. Since they don't have a primary problem with physicians, they should be admitted under orthopedics or vascular surgery."

I replied back 'Sir, this patient will be operated on and then will require a long stay. Don't you think after the operation the major care is under the supervision of a physician? And if it is medicolegal, then by putting my name in the admitting doctor, I am ok with court summons."

He still did not agree. So I called the superiors, but the answer was" We have delegated the admission protocols to Dr. Milind, and we cannot interfere. And sir, what's wrong with them being admitted under other specialties? They will refer to you if needed."

I said, "First thing, having my name on paper will help my patient in all aspects. Counseling, paper work, and future medical and legal help. Secondly, I am not going to operate. So why are you worried?

Still, it looked like they had made up their minds. So I asked them, "Is this true for all consultants?" Because before going there, I have taken data on the last few such admissions.

The answer that they gave shocked me "Dr, you mind your own business. Don't teach us protocols. As of now, you will have to transfer them to someone."

So I refused and came down. I talked to relatives, and all four were shifted to a nearby hospital.

Dr. Desai" But baba, even if you had admitted them under our good friend Dr. R. Shah, you would have been referred."

I said, "I know, but the last answer showed their intent. They had no respect for my bringing so many patients here. Do you know they would lose as much as Rs. 20 to Rs. 25 lakh because of this? All four required multiple surgeries and a long stay."

Dr. Desai" See, this is what I call a sword. You think they lost money. But these are just managers who get their salaries. The loss is the owner's. And what they will do is project you in a bad light with all the stakeholders. So it is you who lost in this hospital".

I knew he was telling the truth in a way. But I felt these managers were not here to dictate terms but to ease the process. And over and above that, there have to be the same guidelines for all.

So that's Dr. Desai for you. He had a practical head on his shoulder and an analytical mind that he used before any actions. And here I am, who speaks first and then thinks later. Or if I can say who has a sword ready for anything I feel is wrong and should be protested against. On a longer run, I always remained at loggerhead with almost every manager that came to this hospital. I have one line for this situation that I psychologically used to give myself a boost "This manager will come and go, but I will be here till they say get out."

Then another one in the team was Dr. R. Shah. He was the Orthopaedician. He was older than me. I always say to him that none of the sins of healthcare upgrading have touched him to date. A complete ethical, moral, clinically sound, and safe hand as a surgeon.

One day, while sitting in the lounge, we were all waiting for him to come. He had said that he has only one patient left to consult, so he will be there. So we thought, let him come, and then we will order our daily tea.

Dr. U.Shah" This is ridiculous. This man has taken almost 30 minutes. He has only one patient, and though he is an orthopaedician, it has taken so long to finish the consultation."

I said, "What do you mean that he is an orthopaedician?

He said, "Doctor, as such, the longer consultations are with physicians and OB-GYNs." Physicians have to ask so many things, write so many things, advise so many things, and then counsel for so many things."

Dr.Desai "And what about the gynecologists?

He said, "See, you have to also ask so many things, examine a lot, and that too in a proper environment, and then give advice a lot."

He continued "An orthopaedician has to just see the history of injury or damage. Their x-rays and other reports are fixed. So he should have just listened and come here for tea."

Actually, we were all really irritated, as we wanted that one tea of the morning very badly. After long OPD hours and seeing so many different patients, we all wanted to refresh with that one cup. And this fellow was making us wait.

So finally, after 40 minutes, he emerged. Dr. U.Shah shouted "Bro, you are actually an MD and MS Orthopaedician. You are more of a physician and less of a surgeon. You counsel so much that patients will get confused about whether to get operated on or not."

We all laughed. Dr. R. Shah said, "But you've known me since college days. I like to be very particular. A complete history, examination, and advice are important."

Dr. U.Shah "Arey, what examination? You have to just say, get an x-ray and bring it back to me. Then, seeing the x-ray, you say you require surgery. This is what almost all orthopaedician are doing. Who cares if knee or hip replacements can wait or not?

He said, "What are you talking about? You have known me for so many years. Just because you are hypoglycemic and require tea urgently does not mean you talk irrelevantly. Stop this or else I will refer you to Dr. Jain."

All laughed at the mention of Dr. Jain. But we all knew how clinical Dr. Shah was. He will not advise operations until he is sure of their benefits. He always said, "If I can preserve the natural joint, then it should be my first priority".

He always took a holistic approach. He will see if the patient could wait for surgery or not, if there is an alternate option, and if the patient is ready to wait or not. Then he will explain everything—diet, exercise, and medicine. He will write down everything in a proper format. He will wait until patients and relatives are finished with their questioning. So Dr. U. Shah was right in saying that he was more of an MD than an MS.

Dr. Desai" We require at least one like him in the city whom we can send our patient. By sending a patient to him, our respect increases".

I said, "Yes, they will always come back or ring and say, "Dr., thanks for referring to such a wonderful doctor. He explained it so nicely."

But again, he was never in the good books of managers.

Dr.Desai "Dr. Shah, you are of no financial benefit to this hospital. Why would you be a favorite of managers?"

I said, "Why are you saying that? He is the best orthopaedician that we can have. Do you know every doctor in this hospital and around, and even the topmost manager brings their relatives to him only?"

Dr.Desai" Ask him how many of the same doctors and managers refer the other patients to him for surgery."

Dr. R.Shah knew that it was right. I asked, "Sir, is this right?"

He said, "Yes, he is right. These doctors and managers want the right advice for their relatives. So they sent them to me. But since I am not pro-surgery in all conditions, they don't send the other patients to me."

I said, "But if the patient requires surgery, then can they send it to you? You're the safest hand, too."

He laughed and said, "Dr. Many times I have said no to surgery for those patients, too. If they are sent for surgery, I don't do surgeries without an examination. So if I feel a patient can wait for surgery, then I advise medical management."

Hearing this, I was surprised. In this corporate world, there was a doctor who was practicing the right kind of medicine, but his own colleagues were not supporting him.

Then one day I came to know about his another part of life. He was settled in London and practicing orthopaedics there. That in itself is a big thing. He had a daughter, and I guess no one will think of leaving such a nice career and future.

So I asked him, "Sir, that's unusual. I have come across only one such doctor who left the roaring practice to shift to Ahmedabad or let's say India. That was Dr. Joshi's finest neurologist one can have around."

I asked, "Why did you come back?

He said, "See, I have a brother who is a urologist and is settled in the USA. My father was a leading pediatrician in the city. He and my mother were alone over here, so there has to be someone. So I chose to come back."

Dr. U.Shah "Dr., why are you forgetting me? Since I came back, you got jealous, and so you shifted back to have a good and drunk life with me."

We laughed. He continued " In the UK, there was a clinical way to practice. You need to be very thorough and updated. Every step of yours is audited. So I kept the same practice for her. I am accountable for my patients' health. They come here with the trust that I will do the right thing for them."

Then there was a final member in the team of four musketeers, Dr. U. Shah. He was the senior ophthalmologist. But when you meet him, it appears he has yet to cross the 16-year-old charm barrier. He was always in a good mood. We always told him that he should not come drunk on weekdays. And he used to shout,"You people have created a bad impression of me in front of all. I don't drink regularly. I only have one or two pegs on weekends."

Dr.Desai" Don't lie. Your voice is slurring, and there is puffiness below your eyes. And it is Wednesday."

He would shout loudly "First of all, Dr. Desai, you are a gynecologist, so don't see things that are not in your expertise. Secondly, I have not slept well at night, and so there is puffiness."

I would then intervene "Sir, but Dr.Desai is a good MD gynecologist. His observation is right on. I am also sure that yesterday you took a lot of pegs."

He would again shout, "Dr. Your diagnosis is wrong. It's possible that my thyroid is not functioning well."

Dr. Shah would then joke "See, two things are in favor of the fact that you were drunk yesterday. Two eminent consultants have seen puffy faces and slurred speech. Second, you are talking irrelevantly by saying thyroid and all."

Including Dr. U. Shah, all laughed.

I asked, "Sir, why are you at loggerheads with the chief medical administrator, Dr. Khatri? He wants your department to expand. Let him. It will benefit you."

He said it, in fact, loudly (loudness was his forte). His voice pitch becomes louder with every word, just like a symphony.

"He does not know a single thing about ophthalmology. In a corporate hospital, you can never have an ophthalmic department where operations are performed."

I asked "Why?"

He said, now very excited as it was his expertise, "See, eyes are very sensitive special organs. We have to be very careful."

Suddenly Dr. Shah shouted, "Oh boss, what do you mean? Your eyes are sensitive, and what we do is not. My work on joints, bones, and the spine is not sensitive.

I also shouted, "What about my working on the brain, stomach, heart, and liver, are that not sensitive?"

Dr. Desai" What are you talking about, Dr. Opthalmo? My branch brings so many new lives on earth, and still it is not a sensitive branch?"

We all laughed. He said with very loud cuss words, "Don't interrupt me. So we require a complete separate set-up with a dedicated, clean operation theater. Out of 10 eyes, if even one complication happens, the government will close down the whole setup. And above all, there will be bad publicity as the patient may lose the eye."

Dr. Shah" Then why do you do such bad surgeries? I never thought you would be a bad surgeon. You are a blot on our friendship."

We laughed, but Dr. U. Shah's next lines were full of local cuss words.

We laughed more. Then he continued" Our hospital has operation theaters for other specialties. If we are to operate there for the eyes, then the chances of infection will be high".

Dr.Desai" But then why is Dr. Khatri not listening to you?

Dr. U. Shah" It is not like he is not listening. But maybe the owners are forcing him. But I guess finally he will agree."

Dr.Desai" You all have problems with management."

I said, "It appears you are the only person in a good book of management. Is there any quid pro quo between you and them?"

Dr. Desai ignored this comment of mine and said, "I can understand why Dr. Shah came back from London. But why the hell did you come back from Bahrain? You and Madam were settled and earning a lot. Why did you come back, and why did you come and meet us only?"

Dr.Shah" Do you know he was the doctor of the Shaikh over there? They met every weekend and enjoyed it." He blinked at all of us. I said "I doubt it, sir. This man will drink two pegs and then start singing in his beautiful voice. I think there will be one hell of a laughter show over there."

Dr.Opthalmo "Boss, at least I drink the alcohol. I am not like you, who flush the costliest and best thing in the world down the toilet. Who does that? You should be sent to jail, or, let's say in Bahraini, you should be made to stand at the crossroads and beaten by whips 1,000 times. And then you should be drowned in an alcohol pond."

It appeared as if all three were visualizing the scene of my bare, obese body being beaten by a whip and then me drowning in alcohol. I shuddered at the thought. But there was loud laughter all around.

Dr. Desai" I heard that you purchased gold and silver yesterday."

He said, "Who is spreading such nonsense rumors? I am completely out of work. I don't have money like you.

I said, "Dr., do you know that one day when we went to his house, I used his toilet? I was surprised to see that all his toilet accessories, like the flush, washbasin, shower, water tap, and even mirror frames and walls, are made of gold and silver."

He laughed but still sent a barrage of cuss words across me. He said, "Boss, you are again spreading lies for me. I don't have cash for all this. Just yesterday I went to deposit cash in the bank."

All three were surprised. Dr. Shah shouted, "Arey, who will go and deposit cash in the bank? Your hard-earned money will now be taken by the government in the form of tax."

We all looked surprised at him. He said, "But I need to deposit some cash in the bank. Otherwise, my whole year's income will appear zero."

Now we are more surprised. We tried finding his cash amount, but he changed the topic.

Just then, Dr. Solanki came. He asked Dr. U. Shah about the patient he had referred. Dr. U.Shah said, "Dr., the patient has a different diagnosis than what you and Dr. Jain are treating."

Dr.Solanki "Sir, but you were referred only for fundoscopy. How come you know the diagnosis?"

Dr. Shah" Do you know whom you are talking to? This man is a complete ophthalmologist. He sees through the eyes of the patient and can see deep inside. If you refer him, you will not require an MRI or CT scan."

We all laughed. But on a serious note, it was a fact that Dr. Opthalmo was the finest ophthalmologist in the state. Whatever expertise he had, he was confident and always right. Dr. Desai" Dr. Solanki, this man is a genius. His diagnoses are always bang on."

Dr. Solanki said "Dr. Jain was not ready to accept your diagnosis. We had an argument, but you know how stubborn he is. But then we went for a second opinion. Even that fellow said your diagnosis Sir, you are great. You saved a patient from delayed recovery and lots of expenses."

Dr. Shah "In that case, let's send the bill for the next three months of our tea and snacks to him. Let him pay as a good-will gesture. And tell Dr. Jain never to take a panga with Dr. U. Shah."

Dr. Desai" It is very nice of him that he has not started a neurology clinic; otherwise, Dr. Jain would have been retired long ago."

We all had a healthy laugh.

I said, "Sir, this man is trying to create a rift between you and your Guru, Dr. Jain. We all know how you always go to greet him especially.

Dr. Shah" Let us tell Dr. Jain that he is thinking of competing with him in neurology. He has started giving expert advice and second opinions to his patients."

Dr. Desai" I don't know about anything else, but the security guard will tomorrow stop Dr. U.Shah and say you are not allowed in this hospital."

We all laughed, but even in this gossip, we know how few of the consultants were the most powerful in this hospital. If they wished, they would make many consultants lives difficult. In fact, indirectly, it was done almost daily.

So here was my group, called Nukkad. All this years I found solace with them. The three had a different outlook on careers, corporate hospitals, management, and even life. These different versions helped verify and correct my version.

In the beginning, we were known in Nukkad as NAVRI Praja, which means "No Work Group." But as we four became famous for our gossip, chitchats, and Masti, many started coming to the doctor's lounge. So after a due process, we christened it with a new name, Nukkad," which means a corner place on a road where all meet to gossip and have tea.

This nukkad helped me keep a sane mind while going through the lean patch of the COVID pandemic. My family was a pillar stone that gave me support, and this Nukkad was another pillar that kept me mentally strong. During COVID, I became part of media debates and became a writer as well. So I made new friends in the form of journalists.

We Doctors Are Criminals For The Larger Society. But Why?

One day, four to 5 journalist friends from different media outlets were sitting around at a Sunday get-together. The topic revolved around corporate hospitals.

I said, "You people are very anti-doctors. You keep blaming doctors for all problems in healthcare."

Mr. Kshatriya" But sir, isn't it true? People come to the doctor with trust. When they get expensive treatment, wrong treatment, or bad behavior in the hospital, they will only blame doctors."

Mr. Golani" And sir, I don't understand why doctors are so money-minded. How much money is enough for doctors?"

I said, "See, partly you are right, and partly the situations have changed."

All of them turned their eyes toward me. So one of them asked, "What do you mean?"

I said, "Suppose you go to your doctor in his clinic, then what happens? So you meet him directly, or there are roadblocks?"

Mr. Patel "Sir, when I go to my doctor, I sit in his reception. Then the doctor calls me, sees me, and gives me a prescription. Then I go out, pay the amount, and leave."

So I said, "You directly deal with the doctor and the receptionist and pay as per his fees."

They all agreed.

Then I asked, "When you admit yourself to a nursing home, what is the scene of doctor consultation, treatment, and billing?"

Mr. Vyas" We talk directly to the doctor; he admits, he manages, and then he gives us a bill."

I said, "So correct me if I am wrong that you have direct access to the doctor, and even in billing, the payment, adjustments, and discounts are smooth."

All said yes.

I "Mr. Golani, when you came to ASHA last week, do you think it was smooth?"

Mr. Golani "Oh, doctor, it was like going to meet a big-shot politician, or an actor, or a beaurocrats."

I asked "Why".

He said "They made me sit outside your room. Then they made me fill out a form, though I told them I was meeting socially with you. Then they gave me a voucher to go and pay the fees.

Then, as you intervened, these things were canceled, and I met you. When I came out, I thought I could go out now, but I was stopped and a feedback form was asked to be filled out. And then I left."

I asked, "Mr. Vyas, last month one of your relatives was admitted, and then I remember you rang me for various complaints."

He said" Yes. They were admitted under the care of a surgeon for an operation. The surgeon was known to the patient, and so he has told the relatives to go and admit her to the ASHA hospital. They went, but they were made to stand in a queue for an hour. After filling out the forms and various other formalities, they were asked to deposit Rs. 50.000. When they said they had a medical claim, the counter told them they still had to deposit."

So they called the doctor. He talked to the admissions counter and asked them not to take deposits from the patient. The person said, "Sir, if you are saying we will not take it, then you need to sign the form, and the responsibility will be yours if a payment issue happens."

The surgeon was angry; he said, "Boss, I am the leading surgeon in this hospital, and I have already told the manager that this patient is my relative. Still, they are being harassed like this."

The person was blunt "Sir, I know you, but this is what we are being told to do. We are following the rules. And sir, this happens to all the patients."

I asked, "So then the surgery was smooth, I guess. What happened during the stay?"

He said, "The patient and the relatives felt like they were in jail. The home food was not allowed. The patient's food was pathetic. And when the relatives said they would bring food from home, they were refused. Even when the surgeon said to allow it, he was told that it is against hospital policy".

I asked, "What happened during discharge? Was that smooth and early?"

He said, "Once the doctor discharged me, it took me 10 hours to be released. The billing was a big harassment. The bill was completely in an alien language. The heads in the bill were like service tax, nursing charges, infusion charges, drug dispensing charges, and what not."

I asked, "What about the surgeon's charges?

He said, "It was around 5 percent of the total bill."

I then turned to Mr. Kshatriya and asked, "When your father got admitted to a nursing home, how was the process?"

He said, "We got the bed the moment I reached the hospital. The forms were filled out in my room. I brought my food and medicines from outside. And for any issue, you and the other doctor were available in cabins every time. And during billing, it was hardly half an hour. So I guess smooth."

I asked Mr. Golani, "See, this is the difference. In corporate hospitals, between me and the patient, there are managers, formalities, and rules."

Mr. Patel" But then, sir, we get all the facilities in the corporate hospital. The food of the patients, medicines directly from the hospital, and cashless facilities. Even the big machines are available. And all specialties are there under one roof."

I said, "Exactly my point. If you say you are going to a corporate hospital for this reason, then if it is costly, it is not because of the doctor. We are also hand-tied. Still, none of you have ever said that the businessmen running the hospital are looters".

Mr. Kshatriya" But sir, when you know this is the problem, then why do you go there?"

I smiled" When a patient was ready to accept certain shortcomings of nursing homes like food, medicines, and fewer facilities, we were happy to have nursing homes. But now that you people want luxury, facilities, central AC, and all things under the roof, these corporate hospitals have increased. And then cashless facilities and all specialties under one roof are also requested by patients."

I also said, "Along with this, we as doctors don't have this much money to make such big hospitals or invest in such big machines. So to upgrade our expertise and decrease compromise in management, we also get attachments to the hospitals."

Mr. Golani" But sir, I agree with what you said. But then what about the nexus of doctors with hospitals and pharmaceutical companies?"

Mr. Kshatriya" It is not that only businessmen are looting. They cannot do this without the help of doctors. The extra reports, high-cost medicines, extra stays in the hospital, and unnecessary procedures are advised by doctors only."

I said, "So again, you are right. I agree that with the increase in corporate culture, doctors are ready to do what the managers tell them to do. They want to be in the good books of managers and the marketing team of hospitals. So that they get more patients."

So I guess my arguments fall apart with this last question of theirs. Mr. Golani said that day "Sir, there are definitely many doctors who are good and ethical. But that line of demarcation is getting blurred. So if you feel that only businessmen are wrong, then it is half the truth. They can build hospitals and invest in big machines. But for profit, if they want something to be done, then that blood is in the hands of doctors. You can't defend that."

I Never Thought About Such Changes In Corporate Culture. This Is A Definite Self-Destruction Mode.

As the years of my practice went by, many managers changed in the hospital. Finally, a day came when the original owner sold the whole stake to an investor firm. Till now, almost every hospital in the city has had a thorough corporate culture. They had a full-time culture in their hospital. The doctors were working full-time and only in that hospital. Even they were made to stop their private clinic.

But at ASHA Hospital, almost 95 percent of doctors were honorary, had private practices, and also practiced in other hospitals. So still, this hospital thrived on patients who came to see only particular consultants. These consultants were so reputed that they were part of policymaking, consultants to big politicians, governors, and professors of the majority of doctors during their residency days. Even so, there were few who were awarded the nation's highest civilian awards. Out of 5 consultants who were in the COVID task force that formed policy for Gujarat state, 3 belonged to ASHA hospitals.

So when the new management came, they started showing their intent to make this hospital a full-time culture. The resistance came from every corner. These consultants had one principal in their lives, and that was, "We will never be slaves of any hospital. We will serve patients and not hospitals.

Dr. A. Patel" Dr. Gupta, these people have brought a drug formulary. Now they will decide which brand will be given to the patients."

I said" Oh. But then, that was done previously as well. I guess only a few consultants were asked about their brands; otherwise, the purchase department made a policy of drug formularies."

He said, "Yes, you are right. But that was actually made by consultants, whom we know are best at deciding the quality of medicine".

I said, "Yes that I agree".

At least we knew Dr. Patel, who was the head of that committee along with Dr. M. Patel.

He said" Yes. Because of this, we got proper standards and good-quality brands for our patients."

"So now what are they planning? I asked

Dr. Joshi "See, I am a surgeon, and so I don't understand these brands and all. But still, if they are going to bring substandard brands, then our patients will suffer. Why are they doing so?"

Dr. Rawal" They are doing this to increase their profit margin."

I asked, "What is that to do with profit margin?"

Actually, on that day, we had no idea about this drug formulary issue. But soon I came to know. I was called one day to be part of the drug formulary team. When I went to the conference room, there was a MD (Managing Director) of the hospital, a ZD (Zonal Director) of the hospital, the purchasing head of the whole group of hospitals, and four doctors of different fields. Along with this, we were connected with all four hospitals in different cities. We have hospitals in Ahmedabad, Vadodara, Rajkot, and Gandhidham. So in all, almost 30 to 35 people were connected.

The meeting started.

The purchasing head took over and said, "Sir, we have seen the different drug formularies of all hospitals. We saw that there were many brands for the same molecule in all hospitals."

He continued" So what happened was that, though we had bulk power, different brands led to the belief that we had less volume. But the volume of molecules is huge."

I was getting to what he was trying to explain.

So the ZD said, "Now suppose if we make our drug formulary uniform, then what will happen is that in one molecule we can have only three brands. Now with this data, we can talk to companies to get the best deal for bulk purchases."

Until this, we were in agreement. This served the business purpose as well, and till now there has been no talk of compromise in the quality of the medicine.

But then the bombshell came. The purchase head continued. He then showed various examples of common medicines. He showed which brands they were negotiating with.

The cardiologist, the physician in Baroda, and the orthopaedic surgeon in Rajkot shouted, "Sir, the brands you are showing to us are very substandard and local brands. We have not heard these names either."

Still, the purchase head continued "Sir, if they are making products, it means the licensing authority has checked the quality."

I was shocked to hear such arguments from a purchasing head. If he is appointed to such a big hospital group, he needs to know the facts about the industry "Sir, then why do you need a drug formulary committee of doctors? If you and your industry are so sure about the quality, then do as you like."

The MD intervened" No, sir. It's not his intention to oppose you. But he is just making a point. It is our understanding that it is the work of authorities to check for good-quality medicine."

A doctor from Rajkot intervened" Then let's have generic medicine only in our hospital. They are also made in our country, so we know they are also of good quality."

One of them went much further when he said, "We will know when some relatives of management are admitted here and they are given such substandard medicines."

The ZD of that city was angered by such a comment, and he said, "Doctor, this is below the belt.

The doctor said, "What about the life of the patient? We all know why doctors are on such committees nowadays."

It appeared the meeting was going south. But still, doctors are known to be blunt. So he continued" You want a signature on paper, and your minutes of the meeting will show that so many doctors were present when this formulary was approved. So if something happens or if the media creates ruckus, you will conveniently tell them that doctors were ok with that".

The MD knew this was bad, so he said, "Doctor, no one is going to blame you. But still hear us out."

So now he has taken over the meeting. He gave a long explanation.

"Sir, we are a hospital that also has to make a profit to run it efficiently. So we are going to have three brands per molecule. One will be a quality, well-known brand, or innovative product. Another will be a low-cost brand that is quality but still cheap. And third will be a mid-section brand, the cost of which will be between them. In the third brand, we can have your suggestions to accommodate according to your volume of patients."

I said, "You mean a doctor who is doing more work here or the head of that department will be given preference?

I laughed and said to myself," A well-thought-out divide and rule policy. The people who work more are the ones who resist more. So if they are taken care of, who else will resist?"

So then, after an hour of heated exchanges, everyone asked to send the proposed formulary, whereby they could make the comments or remarks in that"

After a few days, we all got a mail that had an excel file of molecules with brands. I had been in healthcare for a long time and had made friends with various distributors and purchasing heads in the town. I also had a good friend who, once upon a time, was the head of this hospital. In fact, he was the person who laid the foundation stone for such a formulary.

I sent the Excel to him to get a clear picture. I could see many new brands that I had never heard of. Even when I went on Google to find their location and foundation year, I was shocked to see that many were local brands with no experience, and they depended on third-party manufacturing.

That day, when I got the actual Excel review from Mr. Vyas, I went to meet him.

I said" How r u? It looks like our hospital is going to become a den of substandard medicines."

He said, "Sir, substandard is still ok. But this is absurd. Even the manufacturers of these brands will not take their own medicine if they fall sick."

The statement shocked me. I asked what the moral of the story was.

He said, "Sir, if you see the Excel, they have adopted a theory called high MRP, low cost."

I asked with surprise" Means."

Sir, let me explain by telling you a story first. He said, "This is when I was purchase head of this hospital. We presented a data sheet to our owner showing that there was a molecule that was used in the highest quantity in all our hospitals across the state."

He continued" That molecule was injection meropenem." It is given as an antibiotic and is higher on the ladder of this group of drugs. In the last few years, it has been used by all specialties. So the bulk has increased.

The owner asked, "So. Then we should be making a handsome profit."

Mr. Vyas said, "Sir, we are making money, but we can make many more folds of profit if we see this sheet."

He said, "Sir, last year we allowed one brand to enter our hospital as they were ready to give it to us at a low cost. The MRP was high, and we got it at a low cost, so the margin of profit was higher. So we estimated that if this molecule is written at the same rate, then through this brand we will earn more."

The owner was all ears now. Mr. Vyas continued "Sir, now what I am proposing is that all the leading doctors will listen to you as you have helped them establish their careers from inception".

The owner laughed and said, "Yes, they will. They were nothing when I started supporting them. And now they are all leading consultants for the state. Many have even gotten bungalows, cars, and awards because of the platform we provided."

Mr. Vyas" Yes sir. So if we get a company that can manufacture this molecule for us only at the MRP we want, then our profit margin will be many fold. So let's say we give an order of 10,000 vials, the MRP is kept at Rs 4800 (at par with existing available brands), and our purchase cost is somewhere around Rs 120, then yearly we can make anywhere around 4 to 5 crores."

The owner "In a single molecule?"

He said, "Yes."

The owner got greedy and said, "Then why don't we do this for as many brands as possible? These doctors will do what we tell them."

Mr. Vyas" If I may suggest, let's start a pilot project with this molecule, and once we see it working, we will replicate."

The owner looked miffed, but he knew Mr. Vyas was right.

Mr. Vyas told me, "So that's the story of high MRP, low cost."

I said, "Ok, so this new management is getting these drugs manufactured for themselves?"

He said, "No sir. Nowadays, that is not required. If you have a bulk order and are ready to pay in advance, then you get good negotiating prices."

I "Means by unifying the formulary, they are actually getting a bulk quantity. With that quantity, they will negotiate with companies for a better price."

I laughed. Mr. Vyas asked, "Why are you laughing, sir?"

I said, "Mr. Vyas, just to clarify, I actually knew about the bulk purchases by you people in those days. But can you tell me the end of that story? What happened to that bulk? Why did you not carry on with the full-fledged plan in all other molecules?"

He said, "Sir, we got the bulk of 20,000 vials. The owner said we would try to finish this in a year and a half. He was sure doctors would write."

He continued" But after 2 years, we have to dispose of almost 15000 vials, as no one prescribed."

I said, "Do you know why?".

He said, "Sir, we had a meeting with the pharmaceutical and technical committees for this. This was the committee that was established to regularize the drug formulary."

I asked, "Then what happened?"

He said "Sir, the chairman was Dr. Patel sir and Dr. M. Patel sir. They both blasted us left and right. Dr. Patel sir said in that meeting" We might have respect for you and the owner, but we have some ethics left. We have patients through ASHA Hospital. There is no doubt about that. But those patients got better or survived a death scare because we practiced our medicine right. If the quality goes down, then morbidity and mortality increase. And with the increase in suffering and death, who will come to us or to this hospital?

Dr. M. Patel" Since you are the owners, we cannot stop you from purchasing this brand, but we will not recommend it to be used. This company, which has made the brand, has no experience in manufacturing, has no proper certificates of quality assurance, and has no proper trials."

So now I intervened" That's why I laughed. A businessman, a manager, or an MD can have the arrogance to think their doctors will do as they say. But let me tell you a small fact"

Mr. Vyas knew what was coming. He has been with me for a long time and has seen my journey during COVID as well. I was most critical of policymakers, managers, and even doctors. So he listened silently.

I said, "See, we are dependent on corporate hospitals as we cannot afford such big investments. Second, we are dependent on insurance companies and marketing teams as well. But all this is up to that only".

I continued" There might be a few rotten apples who write extra investigations, medicines, or do unnecessary admissions or procedures. But largely, we will never harm our patients. Tell me how many patients around you have been mistreated by doctors. If we were so morally corrupt, then the majority should suffer or die."

The Era Of Migration With A Dream Of Better Managers And Work Cultures.

The next day, we were sitting in the doctor's lounge when this topic came up. One of the senior consultants declared, "I am shifting my practice to another hospital. I will not be coming here until next month".

I asked, "But sir, you have been here since the day it was inaugurated. Now why are you shifting to a new hospital?"

He said, "Here, the management has no vision. They only want to earn money from every corner. There is no sense when they talk about marketing, drug formularies, and quality services."

Dr. Desai" But sir, even the hospital you are going to will have the same managers."

He said, "Agreed, but at least they have accepted my demands."

I asked "Means?"

He said, "See, I am the senior here. I can't work like a junior consultant. I need someone to help me. I have a name in the town, and people come because of my work. But these new managers have declared that my visiting cards and letterheads will not have my mobile number or my email ID".

It was news for us also" But how is that possible? Our mobile number and email ID are the last remaining ways of contact for our patients with us".

He said, "Exactly. In corporate hospitals, both in OPD and indoors, our patients cannot reach us directly. So they meet different managers in between who miscommunicate with them. Having our mobile number helps them at least to ring or send a message."

I said, "But I think there is more to this abuse."

Dr. R. Shah" Means?"

I said, "Sir, they want every patient to ring on a number that will be a hospital number. So for the next follow-up or in the case of a new patient, they will give an appointment. That way, they can ultimately decide who will see the patient. By doing so, our patients will become their database."

The senior consultant said, "Actually, that's the aim of these managers. They want all our hard-earned patient lists in their system. They will call them, they will divert them, and they will lure them to consult only those doctors whom they wish. By this, we will become easily expendable."

Dr. Joshi"Oh, that's so bad. This new breed of managers are creating problems that we never thought. This drug formulary is already creating ripples. We are ok with good brands, but why bring bad brands and harm patients?

I explained to them what I knew through the discussion with Mr. Vyas. All were shocked to hear the story of the bulk purchase by the previous owner. But someone in the team said, "When will these managers realize that doctors may be pressured to an extent, but how will they bring patients to their premises if the patient doesn't get results? If the bill shows such exorbitant prices for medicines and they don't get results, they will change doctors and hospitals. Then if they don't have patients, why will they have bulk purchases, and when they don't have quantity, why will the company negotiate?

I said, "Brother, you are so right. But the managers don't care. Before this situation comes, they would have shifted to another hospital, and then a new manager will come with new management lessons and new ways to earn."

We all laughed. We all know doctors are trapped in this profession. We have our fallacies, but if we look at world data, the majority of patients get well or survive the death threat because of the decisions that a doctor makes. His clinical acumen, his knowledge about the right investigations and their interpretations, the right medicines, and then knowing the duration of the care are what make a patient better.

Doctors are the ones who decide everything about a patient, but when managers and business principles decide what the doctor needs to investigate or prescribe, or if they tinker around with these decisions, then the real sufferer is the patient.

Policymakers Have No Knowledge About Medical Practice. They Only Know How To Order.

"Dr. R. Shah Looks like our practice days are over?"

"Dr. Desai" Sir, if you feel old enough to retire, then do retire, but why say this type of thing? We have so many years of practice left. Our kids are also small."

Dr. Shah" Doctor, have you read the new order of the National Medical Council?"

He said, "No."

Dr. Shah "You keep playing video games on your phone."

I "You are right. NMC has now issued another order that is going to cause a complete chaotic situation".

Dr.U. Shah" Oh, and why so?"

Dr. R. Shah" Another primitive person. Why don't you two read the newspaper before starting the day?"

"Sir NMC has asked all doctors to write the generic molecule name on the prescription."

Dr. Desai" So what's new in this? They have been telling this for almost 6 to 8 months. And many started writing also."

I said, "Bro, this time there is something very shocking."

Now all ears were directed towards me.

I continued "This time they have decided to punish. They have said that if someone is found to be writing a brand name or if anyone complains and it is found true, that doctor will be suspended for 1 to 3 months."

Almost both Dr. Desai and Dr. U. Shah loudly spoke many cuss words.

Dr. Desai" What the hell? What power do they have to suspend a practicing doctor for the sin of their government?"

I said, "They have been given that power in their constitutional framework by the government".

Dr. Desai" But if we doctors write generic names, then do all hospitals and pharmacies have those medicines?"

I said, "Doctor, you have not listened properly. We are not going to write generic brand name. We have to write a generic molecule name."

Dr. R. Shah "Means?"

I said, "Sir, what is the generic molecule name of Voveran tablet?"

He said, "Diclofenac sodium."

I asked Dr. Desai, "What is the generic molecule name of Tab Siphene?"

He said, "Clomiphene citrate."

I asked Dr. U. Shah, "Sir, what is the generic molecule of Diamox tablet?"

He said, "Oh, why are you taking exams? I knew this around 30 years ago, in my second "MBBS. But I guess acetazolamide."

I said, "Same way, sorbitrate is isodorbide dinitrite, ganaton od is itopride, alminth is albendezole, and so on".

I said, "Now this order says I need to write this generic molecule name."

Dr. Desai" Oh, that's impossible."

I said, "Exactly."

I continued" When we used to study medicine in MBBS, we used to remember only generic molecule names." So it would have been easier then to write this name on a prescription."

"When we started going to clinics for MDs or any postgraduate field, we were so confused."

Dr. Desai "Yeah, in those days, all doctors or professors used to write brand names. So they were the most dreadful days for us. We knew only generic molecule names, and we were suddenly told to remember thousands of new names as brand names."

I said, "When. I asked the professor, and he said, what can we do? The government only allows brands. So when we also came to clinics for the first time 20 years ago, the situation was the same."

I then asked, "Sir, how do you remember so many brand names? How do I know which are of good quality? We can never find out the manufacturing practices of these companies."

He said then "The rule is simple. You will remember certain names by default as you follow the orders of your professors. Others you will remember as MR will be bombarding you with those names. Many of you will remember as you practice, as then you could see the results this brands give to your patients."

I felt a bit relieved and asked further" But I still don't understand; our curriculum is all full of generic molecules, and the whole practice on patients is full of brand names. Is this not fraud?

He asked, "Partially it is, but please explain how."

I said, "Sir, you are asking doctors who are actually going to treat patients to learn something that will not be available on the market."

I continued" You are allowing thousands and thousands of companies to make brand-name medicine. This company is already creating a corrupt medical industry by luring doctors with gifts. In the name of gifts, they are going to push substandard medicines onto the market. So this is cheating patients who trust doctors and the government for their health."

He said, "I agree. But we doctors in India are destined to be scapegoats for the sins of so many other pillars of healthcare."

I asked, "How and why?"

He said, "We study medicines to treat the patients and provide them with relief from suffering." For this, we are dependent on reports and medicines."

Medicines are produced by a pharmaceutical company. And quality assurance is the responsibility of both the company and the government."

To promote their medicine, these companies have been luring doctors all over the world, more or less. But luckily, that number is hardly 2 to 5 percent."

I said, "Yes, I agree."

He continued" Now the media, patients, a larger section of citizens, and the majority of politicians have painted us as looters, corrupt, and gift seekers."

He said, "As time passes, more and more hospitals are built. These hospitals are owned and run by businessmen and managers. They keep changing protocols to earn more."

While I was narrating all this, Dr. Shah interrupted me. He said, "See how right your sir was."

He said, "NMC, by such orders, forgets that quality is regulated by government bodies. For over a century, patients have relied on doctors. Maybe a few are corrupt, but no one is going to write medicine that does not give results. Otherwise, he or she will lose patients."

Dr. Desai" And sir, if I write a generic molecule, then what has the patient to do to get medicine?"

I said, "The patient will go to the chemist. He will give molecule, generic brand, or branded medicine as per his likings."

Dr. U.Shah" Wow. So absurd. I can bet with you that when the majority of practicing doctors don't know the generic molecule name, then how come chemists know that name?"

I said, "Sir, you are right. What will happen then is that the chemist will decide the medicine's name."

Dr.R.Shah" I am sure the whole distribution logistic has some percentage earnings of MRP."

I said, "You are right, sir. Let say. A drug has an MRP of Rs 100, and a similar drug of another name has an MRP of Rs 200. The margin of the distributor is 7 to 9 percent, and the chemist's margin is 20 to 70 percent of MRP."

Dr. Shah "Oh, on every strip, the price is there for the chemist to earn. So then a chemist will decide the medicine. And these policymakers think these chemists are holier than any human in the world."

I said, "So now a patient is dependent on the pharmacist for quality medicine and the cost of medicine."

We all knew where this was going and how much a patient was going to suffer.

But then Dr. U. Shah said something that punched us. He said, "See, I think this is a good decision for us. Let us all write generic molecule. Do you know what came out of the survey done by the largest newspaper in the country?"

We all asked, "What?"

He said, "More than 90 percent of citizens, educated and uneducated, rich and poor, said that the majority of doctors are corrupt and gift seekers. And more than 85 percent said that this decision is good. How can doctors decide which brand we should take? We, as patients, will decide what is good for us with the help of chemists."

We all saw each other. So I said, "I guess then it is a good decision. If a citizen feels this, that means we are no one in this whole healthcare system. But I think now the judiciary will also take note that all those cases that arise due to failure of treatment due to medicine will have to be dismissed against doctors. Finally, God has listened to doctors like us who have nothing to do with this pharma nexus with doctors."

Though we all knew health literacy was at its lowest in this country, we were shocked to hear that the majority of the patients who were treated well by their own doctors felt that their doctors were corrupt. This level of distrust and misunderstanding is never good for health care. But then we guess a few rotten apples in the fraternity, coupled with the pharmaceutical industry, media, politicians, and judiciary, have created this perception that we are all corrupt doctors. In that case, let the patient, chemist, government, and pharmaceutical companies decide what is right for the patient. We were happy to finally write down what we learned for almost 10 years in college. We never asked this government and system to thrust upon us the brands. None of the students realize this until they reach the clinic for the first time. Finally, good riddance.

The Future Of Healthcare In India That I See

Businessman started investing more in hospitals. They made a protocol of drug formularies, hidden billing heads, full-time slave doctors, and a battery of lawyers.

Pharmaceutical companies kept making substandard medicine unregulated by the government authorities. To sell them, they devised many new formulas that were good enough to trap rotten apples.

Lawyers started enjoying the money they got from filing cases of medical negligence. The judiciary, through various judgments, kept making new guidelines for doctors to follow to avoid these cases. Finally, defensive medicine was practiced in India.

A relative was not happy with the doctor's treatment or answer and beat the doctor to death. Every city and district saw these cases on the rise, and still, the government and judiciary were not in favor of a bill against violence against doctors.

The media was happy to get TRP by shouting loudly that doctors require such thrashing as they are looters and murderers. Their degree should be taken.

The election came, and this businessman running hospitals and pharmaceutical companies gave crores and crores of rupees to party funds.

Finally, medical seats started remaining empty despite the rise in demand for doctors. A day came when, like Australia and Canada, we started importing doctors from China, Kazakhstan, Mauritius, and Vietnam.

A survey was conducted later, and citizens still blamed doctors for not sending their kids to study medicine.

A chief minister of a big state was telling me that soon we will have robots to treat patients, and then there will be no corruption. Who requires human doctors?

Those robots will be run and maintained by engineers and experts in artificial intelligence. Now the judiciary and government have more work to do. They are busy framing laws to implicate this new set of humans for negligence.

A prayer

Indian healthcare is a very diverse subject. Doctors are the starting and ending points, but they are not the policymakers. They remain in the core and try to practice what they have been taught.

A long career in medicine for 30 or more years does count, and with that, let me put forward a few suggestions.

1. Strengthen our medical education. There can be no compromise in studying science that will be utilized to save lives. How can a substandard doctor be allowed to come to the clinic to practice? Make it stringent and use a pyramid system. If you fail, you fall to the ground.

2. Punish the culprits. Accountability is a must in healthcare. Let there be an Indian medical service that, just like the army, governs the doctors. How can a negligent doctor be allowed to practice? How can only monetary punishment suffice?

3. Rural health is a must. But words are not important. A safe and secure environment with a basic healthcare structure and living conditions with a secure future is a must. Nowhere in the world can a human survive for long without decent career security.

4. Pharmaceutical companies. They are pillars of healthcare. How can third-party manufacturing be allowed in this country where quality is at its lowest? We have GST data; find out which gifts were purchased and how many physician samples were manufactured. This will lead to doctors getting benefits. Punish both the company and the doctors.

5. Policy Maker Please appoint those who have practiced medicine. Those who have studied medicine are not good at policymaking. And please keep politicians away from this sector. They are here to provide the resources needed to develop the healthcare infrastructure.

6. Corporate hospitals please regulate them. Don't allow them to make absurd rules that only bring bad names to doctors and healthcare.

Profitability has an upper limit in healthcare. If you want to earn more, go find some other business.

7.   Judiciary Lawyers are needed to get justice and help the needy. But please understand that not all treatment failures are due to negligence. By filing affidavits, you don't lose a single minute of your career, but a doctor loses sleep, career time, and mental strength to continue the good treatment. Don't treat us as criminals for your meager profit. There are repel effects going on in the medical field.

Insurance Don't allow them to make the decision of admission, what treatment is required, and what they will reimburse. When they were allowed to run this business, this was not the understanding. This is fast becoming a reason for distrust between doctors and patients. It is good for a needy patient, but if they are going to charge a hefty premium and still deny it because of hidden conditions, then it is of no use. See where America is today due to this consortium.

About the Author

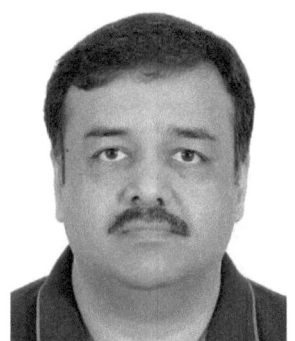

Dr Yogesh A Gupta

Dr Yogesh A Gupta is doctor by profession, a husband and father of 2 beautiful angels. He likes treating patients with all his knowledge at hand. He likes to observe things happening in the medical sector. He is a writer and a speaker. This is his second book that revolves around doctor's journey from college to practice. His first book was based on covid virus. He is husband to beautiful wife and Professor DR GEETA GUPTA. She is a research scientist and a professor in Forensic science. He is father of two beautiful angels MANYA and ARAYNA. This three are support system of the doctor.

He likes to study. Apart from MD Internal medicine degree, he has also got post graduate diploma in hospital management. He is pursuing Post graduate in Medico legal ethics. He has got certificate in AI in healthcare. He is senior consultant physician and Head of Geriatrics. He is also Professor of practice in NFSU.

Right from the study days he has realised the importance of good company. It was group of 8 that help him survive the toughest days of MD internal medicine when he saw worst floods, riots, earth quake and malarial epidemic. It is group of 4" Nukkad Group" that keeps him balanced head during the practice. They 4 keep interacting with each other and upgrade themselves with every changes that are happening around them in medical field.

He presents his second book. Every doctor will relate with the journey. It is for rest others to decide whether they want to see upfront what happens in life of a doctor. Fasten your seat belt.

www.ingramcontent.com/pod-product-compliance
Lightning Source LLC
LaVergne TN
LVHW041945070526
838199LV00051BA/2914